Also available from the American Academy of Pediatrics

Caring for Your Baby
and Young Child
Birth to Age 5*

Caring for Your School-Age
Child
Ages 5 to 12

Caring for Your Teenager

Your Baby's First Year*

Guide to Your Child's Symptoms
Birth Through Adolescence

Guide to Your Child's Sleep
Birth Through Adolescence

Guide to Your Child's Allergies
and Asthma
Breathing Easy and Bringing Up
Healthy, Active Children

Guide to Your Child's Nutrition
Making Peace at the Table and Building
Healthy Eating Habits for Life

New Mother's Guide to
Breastfeeding*

Guide to Toilet Training*

ADHD: A Complete and
Authoritative Guide

Baby & Child Health
The Essential Guide From Birth
to 11 Years

Heading Home With Your
Newborn
From Birth to Reality

Waking Up Dry
A Guide to Help Children Overcome
Bedwetting

Immunizations & Infectious
Diseases
An Informed Parent's Guide

A Parent's Guide to Childhood
Obesity
A Road Map to Health

Less Stress, More Success
A New Approach to Guiding Your
Teen Through College Admissions
and Beyond

A Parent's Guide to Building
Resilience in Children and Teens
Giving Your Child Roots and Wings

The Wonder Years
Helping Your Baby and Young Child
Successfully Negotiate the Major
Developmental Milestones

For more information, visit www.aap.org/bookstore.

*This book is also available in Spanish.

D0048429

Sports Success R_x!

Your Child's Prescription for the Best Experience

How to Maximize Potential AND Minimize Pressure

Paul R. Stricker, MD, FAAP

Sports Medicine Pediatrician and Olympic Physician

American Academy of Pediatrics

DEDICATED TO THE HEALTH OF ALL CHILDREN™

American Academy of Pediatrics Department of Marketing and Publications Staff

Maureen DeRosa, MPA
Director, Department of Marketing and Publications

Mark Grimes
Director, Division of Product Development

Eileen Glasstetter, MS
Manager, Consumer Publishing

Sandi King, MS
Director, Division of Publishing and Production Services

Kate Larson
Manager, Editorial Services

Jason Crase
Editorial Specialist

Theresa Wiener
Manager, Editorial Production

Leesa Levin-Doroba
Manager, Print Production Services

Shannan Martin
Print Production Specialist

Linda Diamond
Manager, Art Direction and Production

Jill Ferguson
Director, Division of Marketing and Sales

Kathleen Juhl
Manager, Consumer Product Marketing and Sales

Cover design by Linda Diamond

Library of Congress Control Number: 2006921056

ISBN-10: 1-58110-227-5
ISBN-13: 978-1-58110-227-7
CB0044

The recommendations in this publication do not indicate an exclusive course of treatment or serve as a standard of medical care. Variations, taking into account individual circumstances, may be appropriate.

Statements and opinions expressed are those of the author and not necessarily those of the American Academy of Pediatrics.

9-152/0506   1 2 3 4 5 6 7 8 9 10

Cheers From the Stands

"A lay publication that appropriately addresses the issues of sports readiness and the healthy involvement of parents in the sports activities of their children has long been overdue. This well-written book hits the mark. It's conversational tone and the logical development of its material makes it a must-read for all parents who wish to successfully introduce their children to the world of organized sports. It imparts the right doses of information about normal growth and development, skill acquisition, training progression, and realistic expectations, and these perfectly dosed bits of information allow the parent to appreciate the complexity of their young, developing athletes. Dr Stricker is to be congratulated on writing a text which is not only easily understood, but also easy for parents to apply to children of any age."

> James C. Puffer, MD
> Former Professor and Chief, Division of Sports Medicine
> Department of Family Medicine
> University of California, Los Angeles (UCLA) School of Medicine

"Dr Stricker provides a unique perspective on the issues surrounding youth sports participation. His focus on how the process of growth and development affects a child's ability to acquire skills, and how this varies among children, is essential information for parents and coaches. Parents of children of all ages will find this book a valuable resource to help guide them in addressing the many questions that can arise as their children embark upon their journey in youth sports."

> John P. DiFiori, MD
> Chief, Division of Sports Medicine
> Department of Family Medicine
> UCLA School of Medicine

"This is an absolute MUST-read for every parent out there. Success is a journey through life, and this book takes us on a great journey helping parents to guide their kids to be the best they can be in life."

Lenny Krayzelburg
Four-time Olympic Gold Medalist in Swimming

"Dr Stricker's expertise combines a unique knowledge of sports medicine with a deep understanding of the pressures associated with the development of our children and sports. This book delivers the necessary education we need to help prepare our children so that their personal performance is optimized at every state of their development. As a mom of 3 young athletes I consider this book to be required reading for any parent, coach, or athletic director."

Genia C. Rogers, MEd
Mother of 3, Business Owner, Public Speaker on Health and Wellness, and Pilates Instructor

"A practical, reality-based approach towards children in sports. A great starting point for parents."

Fred Lammers
Teacher/Aquatics Coach
Santa Ana Unified School District
Orange County High School Teacher of the Year (2005–2006)

To my loving parents Eamil and Paula.

My father left a medical legacy by his example of being a doctor for the sheer passion and love of helping people. Thank you, Dad, for showing me the art of how to serve my patients.

My mother radiates life to those around her. She instills in me the quality to pursue excellence and shares the joy of my every success, big or small. Thank you, Mom, for your gift of undying love, sacrifice, and support for your children. You are truly an amazing mother, and I am your biggest fan!

Table of Contents

Acknowledgments

To my 3 physician brothers, Charles, Wes, and Stephen, who value keeping our family close. Thank you for cheering me on to pursue all the interests of my heart.

To James Puffer, MD, my sports medicine mentor and friend, who inspires me to achieve more than my mind can believe. Thank you and your family for your positive influence on my dreams.

To Coach Robert Pease, who is the coach who changed my life. So much of your belief in me is what continues to provide the fuel and confidence for personal achievement.

To Joseph Wesley, whose support and encouragement keeps me writing. Thank you for helping me not give up on my passion for the youth of our country.

To Ernie Clark, who helped spark this vision into reality. Thank you for that initial defining moment with a visit to the bookstore.

To Fredrik Liljeblad, who cheers loudly and continually. Thank you for having confidence in me and for your many hours of brainstorming, guidance, and wisdom.

Preface

Starting. Running. Jumping. Striding. Sliding. Swimming. Diving. Entry. Pulling. Pushing. Throwing. Tossing. Pitching. Catching. Hopping. Skipping. Landing. Swinging. Accelerating. Following through. Holding. Gripping. Releasing. Grabbing. Bracing. Tumbling. Dancing. Flipping. Twisting. Pointing. Punching. Boxing. Hitting. Blocking. Stepping. Kicking. Tackling. Heading. Scoring. Cheering. Waving. Clapping. Breathing. Panting. Focusing. Psyching. Squinting. Looking. Turning. Hurdling. Skiing. Skating. Spinning. Flying. Twirling. Streamlining. Taping. Bracing. Lacing. Padding. Preparing. Resisting. Lifting. Curling. Pressing. Thrusting. Flexing. Extending. Exploding. Forcing. Exceeding. Yearning. Wanting. Knowing. Leaping. Reaching. Gliding. Blinking. Nodding. Staring. Focusing. Understanding. Pursuing. Visualizing. Yelling. Surfing. Sailing. Practicing. Hiking. Biking. Pedaling. Cycling. Climbing. Descending. Serving. Volleying. Backhand. Forehand. Bumping. Digging. Setting. Spiking. Placement. Rolling. Rushing. Sacking. Defending. Resisting. Exerting. Wishing. Hoping. Pivoting. Shifting. Tensing. Strengthening. Conditioning. Learning. Sparring. Wrestling. Pinning. Vaulting. Rebounding. Dribbling. Planting. Charging. Pivoting. Shooting. Stepping. Passing. Dunking. Stealing. Smiling. Fouling. Supporting. Timing. Sprinting. Enduring. Effort. Accomplishing. Lasting. Losing. Winning. Finishing. Achieving. Improving. Accomplishing. Success.

Warm-up—Get Psyched!

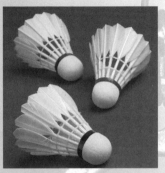

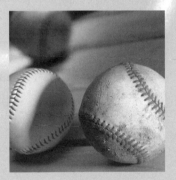

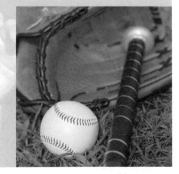

What does *sports success* mean to you? Now that the immediate thoughts have come to mind, I want you to think again. Think hard. What are the things that truly define success for you and your child? Is it the first ball caught without being dropped, or the first-place ribbon? Is it the golden smile after mastering the butterfly, or the gold medal? Is it stepping just right to kick the soccer goal, or is it stepping up on the winner's podium? Please consider these scenarios seriously because how you define success may be how you define your child. If you let society define success for you, your child may come up short. If you have a solid meaning that is a foundational fit for your family, you could save your child's sports life. Success is multifaceted. Success is intimately related to when and how your child develops certain skills, improved body chemistry, and emotional confidence. All of these factors contribute to making your child a more complete athlete for any level of activity.

The progression of skill development can be a beautiful process, like a sculpture, and each level of success is built on the one just before—success is not just the final product.

Youngsters develop sports skills in a sequence, so each sequence should be maxed out for that child. If each developmental stage is fully formed, your active child has the ability to more completely reach her maximum capacity for participation in sports. This leads

INSTANT REPLAY

Success is not just the final product—there can be many successes during the journey.

to a more positive experience and a higher level of achievement, which leads to sports success for your child. Everything returns to how you define—or redefine—success. If success is only the lofty end goal of a gold medal or spot on the Olympic team, that leaves no room for success along the way. What if your child never gets that far? Has there been no success? Let me take this a step further— I want to coin a new phrase for you to embrace called *reality sports success.* When kids are given the opportunity to develop their skills without being pushed, then the reality is that all these kids can have some degree of success with self-achievement and self-improvement!

The bottom line is to be patient. Many young athletes these days are being pushed too quickly through their developmental stages in hopes of early success in sports, only to end up shortchanged. They don't reach their full potential because of pressures to perform. They are robbed. Please don't let a sport *grow* your child; allow your child to *grow into* her sport or activity! This book is a prescription for your child's sports success to maximize performance and minimize pressures to perform. This prescription comes with doses that are easy to swallow. And just like certain medicines, the information here is for your good—all with the intention of a wonderful end result.

Why can't Johnny just come out and play anymore? Our society has changed focus so that now Johnny is urged to come play harder, faster, more intensely, and with pressures to be recruited, make money, secure fame, and head for the pros. Every day I have the privilege to care for other people in my sports medicine clinic. It is a real joy to see youngsters enjoying exercise and all of their different sports activities. It is a pleasure to see parents and coaches with great support and a positive approach toward these young people. On the other hand, it is also stressful to see those kids who are not having fun. When people ask me why on earth I decided to undertake this book, I reply, "Because it is my way to make a house call to the whole country!"

We are in the midst of the terrible "toos." There is too much pressure on young kids and teens to excel in athletics and be the best. Too many youth are trained excessively and get overuse injuries. Too many kids wonder why they are not better than they are. Too many youth have unrealistic expectations placed on them. There is not enough understanding about how kids develop their sports abilities. Not enough information about how kids can succeed. Not enough guidance on how to define success. Too many parents and coaches need and want to know more. This book is written to give them more—more knowledge and understanding of developmental processes—to equip them with information and strategies, all to provide a great sports experience for themselves and multitudes of young people during their quest for sports achievement.

This book will discuss how a child develops sports skills along a sequential path. It will make sense why Johnny cannot catch a Hail Mary pass at 4 years of age. This book will discuss how a child acquires the chemical and physiological means to progress from running 2 miles to 5 miles—and faster than the last time. It will make sense when it is appropriate for Julie to realistically intensify and increase her level and volume of training. This book will discuss how a child's psychological development can affect eventual performance.

It will make sense how to truly support Jermaine during his training and competition. The goal is to help your child avoid getting hurt physically or emotionally or getting burnout from being a little kid overtrained like big adults. Your child will learn that success comes in many different forms besides first and in different colors besides gold. Smiles, everyone, smiles! Sports and exercise should be *fun* for everyone involved and a positive, long-lasting experience.

There will always be pressure to perform. Pressure to succeed. Pressure to win. Pressure to turn pro. Those pressures will not change. What can change is the extra pressure put on your kid today because of unrealistic expectations and a lack of understanding from adults about the process of skill maturation. My heart jumps when I see the joy surrounding the effort of a good performance. My heart breaks when a child's effort is "never good enough," and the hurt shines through the eyes.

I have spent years working with all levels of young athletes, and I want to make a difference that can enable many youth and their parents and coaches to have a positive sports and exercise experience. It is a pleasure to participate on committees and in organizations such as the American Academy of Pediatrics Council on Sports Medicine and Fitness and the American Medical Society for Sports Medicine, both of which advocate safe, healthy exercise and sports for children and teenagers. It has been an honor and privilege to be a team physician for high schools, Division I universities, US national teams, the World University Games, world championships, and ultimately to be selected by the US Olympic Committee to be a member of the US medical staff for the 2000 Sydney Olympic Games—the first pediatrician on a Summer Olympics delegation.

These experiences have granted me tremendous exposure not only to the pressures young athletes face, but also the shared characteristics and experiences that have helped them rise to success.

Sitting on the pool deck at the Olympics brought a realization that "untouchable stars" from the world's point of view were also very real human beings. They were ecstatic about great performances and nervous about their next races; they wanted to see their families and loved ones while trying to forget about school and jobs; they talked about gold medals and television interviews; and they tried to decide if it was the right time to give up their amateur status and turn professional. Some of these conversations were with athletes who were still teenagers. Mere kids. Yet they were also mere budding superstars, flocked by microphones, media appearances, agents, requests from talk show hosts, and calls from the President. All of this is reserved for the recipient of the gold medal—and only the gold. Somehow society has determined that even at the Olympic level, second in the world is not successful. What kind of message is this? It teaches our youth that there can only be a handful of successful people in sports, and in the process sets up the large majority for failure before they even start. I hope this is not how you will choose to define success for your young athlete.

Other scenarios, bad and good, have seared themselves into my memory. Youngsters coming into my sports medicine clinic with overuse injuries from excessive training. Parents looking for a physical cause of their child's inability to perform a certain sport skill. Kids desperately competing to win their parents' attention and affection. Children being pushed entirely too hard at too young an age and being hurt physically and emotionally because they are coached by someone who believes that more is always better. Children pushing themselves too hard because they think it is the only way to be accepted, popular, and successful, falling prey to all the pressures around them. Youngsters finally growing into their sport and happily enjoying success beyond their high school days. Youth whose parents have instilled in them their value and worth outside of their sport. Teens who have persisted for years and finally have a breakthrough performance. Children who love to participate because a coach gives them chances to improve and praises them for their effort, whether they won or lost. Youngsters who excel because they have the support and encouragement from parents who are not over- or under-involved, yet understand the developmental process. Youth and adults who keep sports in perspective. I hope it is obvious that getting second at a world event means many years of previous successes and achievements, and I hope you will be inspired by this book. Please use it to see many ways to help foster years of achievements during those formative years and beyond. Use it to redefine success.

These scenarios are part of my world. They may be part of yours. I became a pediatric and adolescent sports medicine specialist because I love kids, I am an athlete, and I had supportive parents who loved me for me, not because I was a swimmer who won gold. I had a coach whose positive impact was so profound, it helped shape me into an All-American athlete and an adult with self-esteem I may not have had without those years of influence. I was fortunate to be surrounded by people who did things right. I know the world is full of other people who do or want to do things right, too—if they just had the knowledge. Maybe you are one of those people. I sure hope so.

My goal is to make that house call, come into your home, and share my experiences with your family. So build a fire, take off your shoes, pop some popcorn, get comfortable, and pull up your most cozy chair. Let's sit together and talk this over. Let's go over the many developmental processes necessary to achieve and improve in sports and exercise. Once you understand how the pieces fit together, everyone can relax and encourage your child along each stage of the path. Then look out! The sky's the limit for your child to reach his potential—now *that's* success! I want this prescription to be conversational, informative, entertaining, and encouraging so you are happy and eager to let your child come out and play.

★ ★ ★ ★ ★ ★ ★ ★ ★ ★ ★ ★ ★ ★ ★ ★

SUCCESS RX

1. Success is intimately related to when and how your child develops certain skills, improved body chemistry, and emotional confidence.

2. Youngsters develop sports skills in a sequence. If each developmental stage is raised to the full potential for that young athlete, he or she has the ability to maximize per-formance, enjoy a more positive sports experience, and reach a higher level of achievement.

3. Please don't let a sport *grow* your child; allow your child to *grow into* his or her sport or activity.

4. Sports and exercise should be *fun* for everyone involved and become a positive, long-lasting experience.

★ ★ ★ ★ ★ ★ ★ ★ ★ ★ ★ ★ ★ ★ ★ ★

Back to the Future

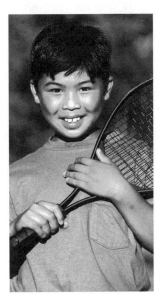

It's a picture-perfect day—warm breeze, sunshine, a day off from school—what more could a kid want? I'm Johnny. My little brother has stopped being a pest long enough to come play with me, and we are actually having fun. Hmm…a big black car just pulled up into our driveway. I think it made a wrong turn. No, it looks like someone's parking the car. I better go inside and let my parents handle this one because I know I'm not in trouble! Hey, maybe they can take my little brother away! Nope, he's really not that bad. I wonder what these guys want, anyway?

Knock knock.

"Who's there?"

"Mr. Agent." Johnny's mom opens the door.

"Mr. Agent?"

"Yes. Can Johnny come play…pro?"

Ah, the low-pressure days of yesteryear. Kids played for fun. Neighborhood children got together and wanted Johnny to come play to even up the teams. They used whatever they could find, mixed together with their wild creativity and make-believe friends, to create a game that was just perfect for them. No fancy outfits, no special gear, just good clean kid fun. Somebody doesn't like the rules? Educate them. The game is not close enough? Change the game so it is. Youngsters are completely capable of making it work.

Ah, the wonders of kids and teenagers learning new skills and having their first successful attempts—the excitement in their eyes, the huge smiles on their faces! They did it! Jamal made his first basket! Julie kicked her first soccer pass! Johnny swam his first lap without stopping! Janie hit her first softball! There is nothing more enlightening than watching children succeed in their own personal triumphs. Youngsters are able to learn games in a positive way.

Moments of the past. Highlights of before. Flashes of history. Fast-forward to today. Wow! What happened? Just like anything else in history, progress brings good and bad. Let's rewind for a moment and be nostalgic. (Get a tissue if you like.) In the 1850s, sports for young children were organized largely through the efforts of the YMCA. These sports efforts spread to public schools in the early 1900s, and the future was set in motion. The Public Schools Athletic League was formed in 1903 in New York to encourage participation by having different categories for variations in skill levels. Unfortunately, organized sports activities for kids basically disappeared in the 1930s because many organizations condemned youth sports, thinking sports activities might be harmful. Youth that were not working found ways to play using sticks and cans. Finally, in the 1960s the heated debates simmered down, leaders came to agreements, and efforts to restore youth sports were made. Changes were made in rules, equipment, and the size of playing areas to acknowledge the limited development and skill levels of children.

Beam me up, Scotty, to the 21st century. How things have changed! Oh, what big muscles you have! The better to finish ahead of you with, sir. Oh, what great equipment you have! The better to win with, sir. Oh, what long hours you train! The better to get a scholarship with, sir. Oh, what wonderful medals you have! The better to be famous with, sir. Win, win, win. First is the only place. Gold is the only color. Winners only come in first. Second is failure. We have gotten a little warped in our thinking. Winning comes in many places, colors, and achievements, and that point *must* be communicated to our children, parents, and coaches.

INSTANT REPLAY

Winning comes in many places, colors, and achievements—and that point *must* be communicated to our children, parents, and coaches!

The feelings that come with winning are a no-brainer. Everyone loves being the best! But everyone cannot be the best, so we have to use every opportunity to help our youth be winners in other ways, too. Reality sports success comes from personal achievement, enjoyment, improvement, and fun. Everything else is a bonus! We must keep the passion and pursuit and get rid of the pride and pressure.

OK, so you want to know what you are getting yourself into with this book. Most people want to know what they can expect. Well, I can tell you, because I know how it ends. This book is a compilation of years of experience as a sports medicine doctor for everyone from grade school beginners to Olympic gold medalists. I have seen young athletes become successful early on and maintain that success, and I have seen youth become burned out or injured and end their careers because they were pushed beyond their physical and mental limits.

There are 4 Ps in the pod of youth sports—*participation, practicality, protection,* and *performance.* The picture being painted in society shows big money and fame associated with sports, and along with that comes huge pressure from unknowing parents and coaches who put unrealistic expectations on children and teenagers. This behavior can cause unnecessary overuse injuries and mental stress from inappropriate and overly intense and zealous training. All youngsters should be allowed to *participate* to learn sports skills, be exposed to many different activities, improve general health, and have fun. Adults should be *practical* and realize that exercise in general is important and not all young athletes can set a world record, no matter how hard they are trained. If you have the knowledge of how youth develop their abilities to be active or play sports, your child can be *protected* from stress and injuries and increase his potential to *perform* at a level that spells accomplishment and reality success for that individual youngster.

This book is divided into 5 sections. Each one describes the progressive interplay between entering a sport and playing a sport and how the development of sports skills is a crucial process in that progression. This information is applicable to recreational sports and exercise as well as organized and competitive sports.

1. *Physical Success.* The first section leads you through the exciting developmental milestones for acquiring skills necessary for different levels of sports from amateur to athlete, baby to baseball, and child to competitor. Information is provided to help adults avoid unrealistic or premature expectations by understanding what happens in the mind and muscle to help Johnny progress from diapers to diving or from spit-up to soccer.

2. *Cellular Success.* The second section describes the details of the chemistry and physiology of the young growing body that contribute to Julie being able to eventually improve her running from 3 blocks to 3 miles. Explanations establish the concept of good foundational training and when increased levels of conditioning become appropriate and productive.

3. *Mental Success.* The third section highlights the maturation processes of the mental and psychological aspects of youth and the effects of these aspects on sports participation, as well as the effects of sports participation on the psyche of your youngster. Tremendous positive effects on self-esteem, self-worth, and sense of accomplishment are prizes of athletics and exercise that are worth more than first place. Concepts of healthy adult support are given to help establish value in your child at an early age when it has the most long-term effect.

4. *Accessories for Success.* The fourth section investigates other pieces of the success puzzle. It discusses the problem of obesity and inactivity in kids, addresses ideas to help avoid common problems, and offers suggestions to produce a successful sports experience. This

section also looks at other aspects of youth sports that can have an effect on sports and exercise, including nutrition and strength training.

5. *Prescription for Success.* The final section brings all of these ingredients for success together to form the right recipe among parent, coach, and child. A prescription is given to help optimize the youth sports situation for everyone involved and allow children to develop and reach their maximum potential.

Now you know what awaits you. So put your feet up, relax, and enjoy. If you have a child, grandchild, or even a future child that might be involved in any sports activities, this book is for you. If you are a parent, coach, teacher, or parent coach, please eagerly read on. Learn new information. Renew old assumptions. Answer more questions. Avoid more confusion. If you think you know everything already, I bet I can surprise you. I want this pediatric house call to help you unravel the kids-sports' mystery of "How to?" into the young athlete marvel of "Can do!"

Just look at the major progress that has been made to provide youngsters with chances to be involved with sports. Within that progress is the change that has allowed more sports for girls, which is now the most rapidly growing group participating in sports. According to the National Council of Youth Sports, more than 38 million youth are involved in at least 1 organized sports activity, with even more kids playing casual sports or being in 2 or more sports. That's a lot of active kids! What a great set of statistics, and such a far cry from the past when kids were not even given an opportunity. At the same time, it should be obvious from these numbers that there will not be more than 38 million kids coming in first place, winning gold medals, getting the best scholarships, going to the Olympics, and turning pro. However, until the rest of the world accepts and understands this fact, there will continue to be those who place tremendous, unnecessary pressure on your child to start younger, train harder, and compete sooner to obtain those very limited prizes.

This is reality. Not reality TV, but reality sports. When you understand skill development, patiently allow skill progression, and encourage achievement and accomplishment, that's reality sports success. Any ribbons or medals are extras.

Excessive pressures often push a young body more than it is able to handle, resulting in an injury caused by overuse. Specifically, *overuse* is significant overload to any tissue in the body. Our bodies are very capable of handling a load, adapting to that load, and then handling a higher load the next time. This body process of microscopic breakdown and buildup is largely unseen. When that process is overwhelmed by stress and loads of effort to which the body cannot adapt before the next event or practice, the breakdown accumulates until there is a noticeable overuse injury, such as a stress fracture of a bone or tendonitis (inflammation of a tendon). Overuse injuries are spoiling the exercise experience. How wonderful that there are millions of kids involved in sports activities; how sad that their fun can be stopped by unnecessary injuries.

INSTANT REPLAY

Excessive pressures often push a young body more than it is able to handle, resulting in an injury caused by overuse.

It is so important for exercise to be promoted positively at all levels and for all kids to be encouraged to be active, whether or not they want to be on a competitive team. Like a good old-fashioned Western movie, there are *The Good, the Bad, and the Ugly.* The good involves the many benefits of exercise and sports participation, such as better fitness, improved body composition, and overall health enhancement. The bad includes the factors that have a negative influence on participation, like competition and sport specialization at younger ages, excessive pressures to perform more at younger ages, emphasis on winning, and training young children like adults. The ugly is what shows up in my clinic—overuse injuries, young bodies and minds overwhelmed by a need to push harder when their bodies can't do it, and kids quitting from burnout.

Overuse injuries are rising in number; I am seeing more and more of these overload injuries every year. Some of these injuries, like stress fractures, were unheard of in children years ago, but now have become relatively common. Stress fractures used to be an adult injury, but that's what we get when we train kids at adult levels. The problem can stem from different causes. Two patients come to mind, both with overuse injuries to the shoulder from doing too much. One child was injured because he was a baseball pitcher and was throwing too many pitches at practice, then throwing many more pitches with dad in the backyard. He was on the local club team, an all-star team, and a traveling team. You do the math. The other child had an overuse injury to her shoulder as well, but it was because she was new on the water polo team, played shortstop in softball, and was learning overhead serves on the volleyball team. These kids both had overuse injuries, but the difference lies in the fact that he did too much of the same sport with his shoulder, while she did too many activities that all involved her shoulder. We have to be aware that overuse is overuse, no matter how it tries to disguise itself. There is nothing wrong with being a good pitcher or involved in multiple sports. However, it is important to realize how easily the body can become overloaded, especially if skill level is being pushed to the limit.

It is difficult to have hard data on the sheer number of injuries caused by overuse because many do not show up in an emergency department, but are treated by athletic trainers, physical therapists, chiropractors, nurses, physicians, or coaches and parents. This makes it possible to only estimate the numbers. Even so, it is estimated that there are millions of injuries of some kind each year that require medical attention and that approximately *half* of those millions are overuse injuries. That is a problem—a big problem. Just because those injuries are associated with sports and exercise doesn't mean they are a good thing. Surveys have shown that parents often feel that injuries are just part of sports, which is partially true for acute fractures, accidents, and plain old bad luck. But overuse injuries should not be seen as routine or even as an athletic badge of courage. It is not healthy for young, growing tissues to be overloaded to the point of meltdown. Aren't you supposed to break in a new car before you drive it too fast? Don't you let your newborn puppy gradually run longer and longer distances with you? Your active child certainly has more value than a car or an animal, so please be sure to treat him that way. This book is about achieving maximum potential, and the athlete machine must be in great working condition for that to happen.

I am not being negative; I am trying to find a way for us to let in some sunshine. I am sure we can all think of a few young athletes who have sustained an injury because of the "overpush" phenomenon from a highly intense coach or parent. You may see it on your child's teams. You may see it in the mirror. Now we can all know better—and do something positive about it.

Overuse injuries should be preventable! Such injuries occur because of many factors, but human error is a biggie if a young athlete is pushed excessively beyond her level of sports skill development. Remember, the focus is on sports skill progression, going from point A to point B. This isn't a game of Twister in which your child just steps from red circle A to yellow square B. Your child grows from point A to point B, and we would all be healthier and happier with the knowledge of how that happens. It is my goal and sincere desire to have a positive effect on reducing the numbers of overuse injuries, stress, and other problems in young athletes who are being pushed excessively. I truly hope you will want to join me.

How far have youth sports come? They've come a long way, and mostly for the better. More opportunities mean more exercise and fitness for our youth, which is extremely important in the midst of an obesity crisis. More participation means more learning of skills that can be applied to many activities, sports, and exercise for a lifetime. These skills are useful to allow young people to try multiple sports instead of learning just one specific skill set. More involvement means more chances to support your child and encourage sports achievements, no matter what level. More time spent enjoying sports activities fosters social skills and friendships and decreases downtime that might be spent getting in trouble.

Unfortunately, though, we have come even further. Younger and younger kids are being pressured by society, media, peers, parents, and coaches. Recruiting pressures were once reserved for colleges, but now even middle schools are recruiting athletes. Rarely does the neighbor come over anymore and ask if Johnny can come play. Too often, the neighbor is Johnny's competition for the starting spot on the fourth-grade soccer team. Gold medal pressures are forcing kids to specialize in one sport at much younger ages, setting them up for adult-type injuries of overuse, sports burnout, and unrealistic expectations. Sensationalism and pressures are allowing many youngsters to think unrealistically that they can be professional athletes out of high school, with fame and fortune as a substitute for education. These collective pressures can overload parents and kids and turn situations into negative sports experiences. It is not enough to just come and play anymore, and it is virtually impossible to stop the pressure snowball that is rapidly approaching. If that's the case, let's find a way to slow it down by understanding how our kids develop. Then positive sports experiences can be the ruling majority, while negative pressures become a smaller minority.

To help cope with the pressures on our youth and keep ourselves from becoming overly stressed, we need to understand the core developmental processes, which will help us stay focused on what's important without distractions from all the surrounding bells, whistles, smoke, and mirrors. See if this plan makes sense—allow your child's early skills to improve, mature, and be refined without being pressured or rushed. When he is able to move on to the next level of development, approach it the same way. Eventually, your child will maximize each stage of development and actually increase his potential for better performance because he will not be rushed through all the stages prematurely. This patience will help your child lay the foundation on which to build as he progressively learns new skills. How exciting! That's what this book is all about.

Most of us are competitive just by human nature—it's part of our primitive survival instincts—but think about this. What is it about society that has allowed us to consider jeopardizing our own children's health for dangling carrots of limited prizes that may or may not happen? Certainly we have progressed far beyond the animals that eat their own young…or have we?

INSTANT REPLAY

If your children are allowed to maximize each stage of development, they will actually increase their potential for better performance because they will not be rushed through the stages prematurely.

★ ★ ★ ★ ★ ★ ★ ★ ★ ★ ★ ★ ★ ★ ★ ★

SUCCESS RX

1. Reality sports success comes from personal achievement, accomplishment, improvement, and fun—everything else is a bonus.

2. Overuse injuries should not be seen as routine or an athletic badge of courage. It is not healthy for young, growing tissues to be overloaded to the point of injuries.

3. Overuse injuries should be preventable.

4. Allow children's early skills to improve, mature, and be refined without being pressured or rushed. This patience will help them lay the foundation on which to build as they progressively learn new skills.

★ ★ ★ ★ ★ ★ ★ ★ ★ ★ ★ ★ ★ ★ ★

Between You and Me

1. Be grateful if your child is able to be active in sports or exercise. How would your life be different if those opportunities were not available?

2. Many adults differ as to why they think their children should be athletes. What are your reasons and motivations behind having your child exercise or participate in sports?

3. It is becoming more important to protect our children from the epidemics of obesity and overuse injuries. How do you portray exercise at home—as a positive lifestyle or as a way to win?

4. Think again about your definition of sports success and the concept of reality sports success. How do achievement and accomplishment play a role in your definition? What preconceived ideas and expectations do you already have as your child becomes more involved in sports activities? How can you define—and now redefine—success?

Physical Success

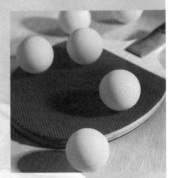

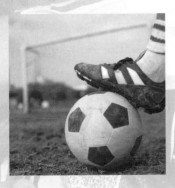

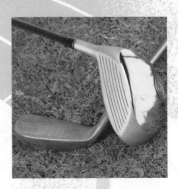

Rome Wasn't Built in a Day

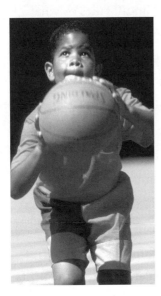

"Ok, kids! Now here's how to do it. Johnny, you stay far to the midfield while the ball is kicked from Julie in the back. She will cut across and then you turn, cross behind, and work the ball to get ready to pass to…"

Wow. I like soccer. It is so fun just running around with everybody. Every now and then I kick the ball if it gets close. Cool shoes, Joey! Just like my awesome blue shoes.

"…as Jermaine sweeps around, he will kick the ball. Then you head the ball to…"

Gee! Look at that hole. I wonder what lives there. Pretty dandelion. I like to blow them when they get fuzzy.

"…the ball gets kicked into the goal. Everybody got it? Remember the play? All right, let's go try it!"

A lizard! Wow, it ran away from me so fast. Uh-oh, everyone is chasing the ball again. What did he say?

One of the first lessons taught to all pediatricians is that children are not small adults. Kids are unique in many ways. We didn't really know we were unique when we were children, did we? We just did what children do—without thinking a lot about rules or what rewards were ahead. Most of us didn't even know what success was until someone made a big deal and told us we had won a game. Lucky for us, but this only lasted for a while.

Kids approach sports from a different viewpoint than adults and gain happiness by mastering skills and accomplishing the previously unaccomplished. Just a reminder—children are *not* small adults. As adults, sometimes we forget that fact and think that if we reason, explain, and demonstrate over and over, a child should then be able to think, analyze, react, and perform like an adult. Not! Of course, there are always exceptions (and by all means, most parents think their child is one) in which certain youth are gifted with talents and abilities outside of what is considered routine for that age. They break the rules of development and cannot be blamed for having exceptional talent. That is fortunate for them, but every other child cannot be expected to keep up with them. The majority of children go through a series of maturational events on their way to accomplishing different sports skills that follow a more routine time clock.

INSTANT REPLAY

Children are *not* small adults.

There are so many different factors that add to the picture of how your child will develop certain skills and be better at some skills than others. Just because youngsters follow a sequence of skill development doesn't mean they develop every skill equally. Thank goodness—how boring would it be if every child was equally good at every skill? That wouldn't be sports; that would just be cloning. Obviously, we must always give credit to genetics. Young athletes can have many equal factors and train exactly the same, yet end up with very different results. I am sure there are children that compete with your child that seem to excel without as much effort. I had a teammate like that in my early years on the swim team. He would miss many practices a week and then find ways to spend the majority of the time getting out of the pool even when he did show up. I rarely missed a practice, I listened intently to my coach, and I worked hard each set to do my best and perfect my swimming technique. When we went to a swimming meet, however, this guy just turned to gold every time he swam a race! He had inborn talent beyond what I had, but he didn't apply it or nurture that talent. Eventually, his performance reached its max because he was not doing the things necessary to improve, and I sadly watched him become pressured and frustrated with the sport. He didn't have reason to celebrate accomplishment because he had done nothing to earn it. Even though I did not win like he did, I had much more reason to feel reality success and accomplishment from my efforts because I was persistent. This consistent persistence eventually paid off as time moved on. I consistently tried to outperform myself, knowing that if I gave my best effort for that particular day or practice, I could accept my performance without

comparing it to the performances of others. I wasn't always happy
with my performance, but I could accept it. All days are not the
same, either. Certain days your child may work hard and not perform
well because of many different factors like fatigue, stress, or illness,
whereas other days your child may work just as hard and perform
out of her mind!

Look at society—we are in the habit of defining successful
performance based on the performance of other competitors instead
of our own effort and performance. If we compare effort and performance to ourselves, we can know when there has been improvement. Let's help your child gain that perspective of reality sports
success. All in all, genetics can be an ultimate factor that separates
even the elite from the other elite, but if each child has the opportunity to develop fully beyond his genetics without as much pressure,
reaching that child's true potential is a successful sports experience.

Set aside genetics. Your child gets what he gets. We have little
control over that, other than to pass our genes down the line. But
there are other variables on the outside and inside of your child
that affect sports skill development and performance over which
you may have a little more control. Outside *(external)* and inside
(internal) factors are very important because they exert complex
influences on sports readiness, performance, and eventual outcome.
External factors include the opportunity to play, local environment
and climate, financial resources, equipment, coaching staff, available
facilities, and safe surroundings to participate. Even if all external
factors could be equalized among youngsters, many athletes
still won't have the same level of ability because of internal factors,

including inherent flexibility, coordination, reaction time, body composition, self-esteem, motivation, heart-lung efficiency, muscle strength, and endurance. Getting a little more complicated, right? This process isn't about picking door number 1 or door number 3, but about mixing different measures of internal and external factors, stirring them with inborn genetics, baking in a supportive environment, and enjoying the aroma as you wait patiently for the finished product.

Just look at every baby book on the shelf. Practically everyone knows when their babies are supposed to roll over, sit up, pull up, and walk. New parents especially memorize every detail of the developmental milestone chart and start saving money for Harvard when their babies beat a milestone by 1 day. (Many of you are smiling right now.) After those milestones, what comes next? Adults track when their children can put 2 words together, dress themselves, tie a shoe, and be potty trained. Ah, but the process does not stop once the kid can flush. The young body keeps passing through developmental planes. Most parents realize that milestones are part of how their children are wired and that it is difficult to greatly change the pattern of how those milestones appear or speed them up beyond a certain point. Unfortunately, parents often do not realize that within the development of sports skills, there are new milestones that continue after the earlier, better known milestones have been achieved. Many often think that once children can walk, they should be able to accomplish any sports skill if they just work at it hard enough or practice it enough times. I don't mean to burst your bubble, but that just isn't the way it usually works.

INSTANT REPLAY

Within the development of sports skills, there are new milestones that continue after the earlier, better known milestones of rolling over, sitting, and walking have been achieved.

Sports skills are acquired in a very progressive sequence.

Sports skills are acquired in a very progressive sequence. Not every child will acquire every skill equally or at the same rate, but most youth acquire them in the same order. So give yourself and your kid a break, just like when she was learning to walk. Pour some tea and learn what exciting things are happening a mile a minute in that cute little bundle of energy you call your child.

During the first 2 years of life, many responses from your child are primarily reflex actions. Touch her cheek and she turns to find food. Touch the ball of the foot and the toes curl over. Touch his hand and his fingers grasp. Proud, beaming fathers of their first-born son already dream of a football star. Stop there. Do not put sand in rattles to make baby dumbbells. Do not install a basketball hoop on the side of the crib. Scientific research tells us that those futile attempts will not work no matter how much you want a head start on Johnny's 3-point shot. Natural curiosity and interaction with the environment will stimulate the growth of motor activity. Close your eyes and think real hard—where does everything go that a baby touches? In its mouth! So be real. Little baby footballs, baseball gloves, and running shoes may be cute and color coordinated, but their effectiveness as sports equipment is lost when they become just another baby chew toy. The American Academy of Pediatrics (AAP) Council on Sports Medicine and Fitness does not recommend infant exercise programs as beneficial for development or helpful for future performance. Supervised, unstructured, and explorative activities in a safe environment are the way to go.

Once children are a few years old, however, hints of sports skill development start to take shape, and the preparation process for sports readiness begins. To be acquired successfully, sports skills involve a complex interaction between movement, sight, and thought. None of these by themselves are completely helpful without the others.

INSTANT REPLAY

To be acquired successfully, sports skills involve a complex interaction between movement, sight, and thought.

Motor skills (movement) require the right visual processing to allow the correct movement response. These skills also require appropriate brain processing and thought patterns so the response will be meaningful and effective. As we go further, you will see that even these processes all mature at different rates during the growth of your child. So let's get started with more specifics and see how different skills for activities, exercise, and sports mature from toddlers to teens.

Motor Activity

Children in the 2- to 5-year-old age group get their motivation and develop motor skills from self-play behaviors. Active games and play in the backyard, with friends at the park, or in heavily padded rooms can provide great sources of exercise in addition to nurturing that important relationship between parent and child. Toddlers and pre-schoolers spend a lot of time just trying to master basic fundamental skills such as running, skipping, kicking, jumping, hopping, catching, and throwing. Kids acquire most of these skills by early elementary school. Adults may not be able to understand that these activities really do take some effort for children. Much of the maturation process of controlling movement in children involves being able to move in different ways without falling over. Obviously, mastering those basic skills is a fundamental step children have to complete before they can proceed much further.

Infants may rely mostly on visual and oral information, but toddlers move away from the mouth being Command Central. They begin to process signals and cues from their brains and inner ears that may even cause a temporary decrease in their ability to maintain good balance as they approach their fourth or fifth birthdays. Children can become overloaded with these signals while walking or running, and they must concentrate just to stay upright. Putting all of their attention into balance control may temporarily interfere with their ability to improve performance in other skills if there are other variables in the environment, such as many other players or uneven playing surfaces. Certainly with time, the act of jumping up and down and running around becomes easier without requiring as much focus to stay vertical. If we could see what is going on in the minds of some young children, it might be very educational. While adults are yelling, "Get the ball! Get the ball!" the child may be thinking, "Don't fall down! Don't fall down!" That is why early soccer teams have been referred to as *beehive* soccer—many players simply swarm and follow the ball just trying to kick it, much to the dismay of the coach, who realizes that none of them are following the instructions of the detailed play outlined just moments before. There is obviously a wide range of abilities in this age group, but relatively few children are really talented at these basic skills. It has been found that fewer than one third of 2- to 5-year-olds are truly effective at throwing and catching.

Visual Ability

Vision is not mature in this age group, and toddlers have difficulty tracking a moving object and figuring out how fast it is speeding toward them. This poor score on visual skills is related to eye movements that are not precise, minor farsightedness, and incomplete development of vision centers in the brain. Hopefully, this information makes it is easier to see why it is difficult for some kids in this age group to hit or catch a moving ball in tennis, basketball, football, softball, baseball, or volleyball, or judge an upcoming wall for a flip turn. It is not simply a lack of coordination or just needing more practice; it is a lack of true visual maturity that is the culprit. Now that age-old phrase of hand-eye coordination finally makes more sense! If 4-year-old Jermaine cannot hit or catch a ball you throw at him in the backyard 100 times, please repeat after me—"Jermaine is *not* a failure at sports." Congratulations and hats off to organizations like Little League baseball that have adapted to make up for the natural deficits at this age with such activities as T-ball. Toddlers and young children can do much better if they are allowed to kick or swing at a stationary ball. Many sports situations would be better for kids if the ball sizes, playing fields, equipment, and practice times were more custom-made for those young learning beings.

INSTANT REPLAY

Toddlers and young children can do much better if they are allowed to kick or swing at a stationary ball because of a natural lack of visual maturity at that age.

Mental Capacity

Toddlers have short attention spans (surprise, surprise). They also focus excessive attention on single items no matter their importance (no kidding!). That is why Johnny may be so distracted by an odd-looking bug or brightly colored flower that he is completely oblivious of a ball or player going by. Periods of instruction should have as few surrounding distractions as possible and are usually most effective when given as show-and-tell. Youngsters require small amounts of information because the proverbial "too much information" can over-load even the most interested toddler in the group. Young children are still concrete thinkers and have difficulty with abstract thinking or processing complex instructions.

Application

Skills are acquired primarily through unstructured play, so active play such as tag should be encouraged. If there is any organized play, it should be very brief, with the majority of time spent having children just playing among themselves. Frequent changes of players should occur to expose children to different positions. Do not keep score. True competition offers no advantage and should be avoided during this age group.

The primary goals of sports activity for toddlers and young children should be playfulness, experimentation, exploration, and having *fun*. Shudder at the thought, I know, but face the facts. Children just begin to develop the intellectual and thinking skills necessary for next-level activities and safety at around ages 5 to 6 years. And if that did not make you gasp, this one will—research shows that participation in sports programs during the toddler years does not seem to give any long-term advantage for future sports performance. Uh-oh, does that mean that spending 3 hours a day practicing with your 4-year-old daughter won't make her a better kindergarten or grade-school athlete? That's right. Specific skills can be refined by repetitive practice only after the right level of motor development has been reached. Basic ground-level activities for children such as walking, running, swimming, tumbling activities in beginner dance and gymnastics, basic soccer, basic martial arts, and skating are suggested appropriate activities. In addition, walking, running, and swimming are activities that also develop fundamental skills that are important for safety throughout life.

These activities can form sturdy foundations for exercise and sports participation on which future skills can be building blocks for the Great Wall of Sports. A few words of caution, however—just because these activities can be started early in life does not mean that these sports should be aggressively pursued early in life. We have all seen Olympic moments showing the rise of sports stars who started

their sport at age 3. But that does not mean they started training sub-
stantially or competing heavily at 3 years of age. These situations are
often misinterpreted by other parents and young athletes because
we don't always know the rest of the story. Those youth later became
Olympians because of many more factors than an early start date, and
research from the US Olympic Committee shows that most Olympians
distinctly point out that they had support from their parents, were
not pressured, and stayed in their sport because of the love of the
sport and because they had fun. Sports activities may be started early
if approached with a non-pressure attitude that focuses only on basic
skills and not with the presumption that this is the beginning of an
Olympic or professional debut.

The benefits of general exercise and sampling many sports along
the way are critical for your child to have the most potentially successful outcome possible. However, some children decide (or their
parents decide for them) to specialize in one certain sport at a very
early age. This practice is actually not supported by the AAP Council
on Sports Medicine and Fitness because of the potential risks from
premature sports specialization. Repetitive actions and long hours of
training can overload the young growing body and cause overuse
injuries such as tendonitis, growth plate injuries, and stress fractures.
As I mentioned at the beginning of the book, overuse injuries are
becoming rampant among our young athletes. The earlier a child
starts to become exclusive with one sport, the sooner she can show
signs of overload. Swimmers are notorious for getting inflammation
of the shoulder because of the high number of arm strokes taken during practice. Kids in throwing sports can stressfully widen the growth

plate of the shoulder or elbow. Gymnasts can overload the growth plate in the wrist, causing it to finish growing prematurely. Sports with repetitive bending or twisting can cause microscopic fractures of the spine. Sing with me—"These are a few of my least favorite things."

Specializing in a sport too early may also lead to lopsided skill development. This may not appear to be a big deal if the child is good at that sport. Yet, if that child is only good at one thing and is then injured or wants to change sports, she will find herself at a deficit. Focusing on only one sport at an early age has its mental cuts and bruises, too. Lack of socialization skills can occur if a child is isolated from her friends and life outside of that sport. If the pressure of competition is emphasized before the child is emotionally ready, the child can become burned out and have to retire from a sport before the teenage years. On the other hand, clearly there are examples of young kids specializing early in sports, having a positive successful outcome, and also transitioning into the rest of society at the end of their sports careers. If only they all could be so lucky.

When children are young, they are a package that is just beginning to be unwrapped! The process is so exciting because you and I cannot predict the final present just by shaking the box. The developmental stages are in motion, so have fun watching your child change. Fun is good for children and adults. Isn't it amazing how much of the developmental process occurs after the Big 3 of rolling over, pulling up, and walking? As more of these sequences are unveiled, it is my desire that we all respect these natural limitations and allow our children to maximize each level along the way to produce the most successful outcome possible!

★ ★ ★ ★ ★ ★ ★ ★ ★ ★ ★ ★ ★ ★ ★ ★ ★

SUCCESS RX

1. Children are not miniature adults and are very unique in many ways.

2. As a society, we are often in the habit of defining success based on the performance of other competitors instead of our own.

3. Sports skill milestones are acquired in a progressive sequence. Not every child will acquire every skill equally or at the same rate, but most youth acquire them in the same order.

4. Toddlers and preschoolers spend a lot of time just trying to master *basic* skills such as running, kicking, hopping, and throwing. They also must concentrate significantly on controlling their balance to stay upright, which can temporarily interfere with their ability to improve other skills.

5. Fewer than one third of 2- to 5-year-olds are truly effective at throwing and catching.

6. Toddlers have difficulty tracking a moving object because of eye movements that are not precise, minor farsightedness, and incomplete development of the brain's vision centers. Understand that this is a *natural* deficit during this age group.

7. Young children have short attention spans and require short periods of show-and-tell instruction.

8. Skills are acquired primarily through unstructured play. The goals of sports activity for toddlers should be playfulness, experimentation, exploration, and fun.

9. There should be no emphasis on competition or premature sports specialization at this age.

★ ★ ★ ★ ★ ★ ★ ★ ★ ★ ★ ★ ★ ★ ★

Between You and Me

1. Think of how your child carries out certain sports skills. Do you see your child's abilities in a slightly different light now?

2. Remember that foundational skills provide the building blocks on which other skills will grow. What basic skills are your child learning now, and how can you avoid rushing their full development?

3. Parental involvement during these early years serves as an important role model. What kind of unstructured play opportunities can you creatively think of to help your toddler use those basic foundational skills he or she is capable of performing while having fun at the same time?

Moth to Butterfly

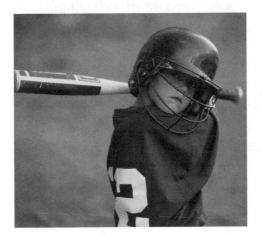

Yea! I kind of like sports this year. I tried some last year, but couldn't always figure them out. Some sports were just too fast for me, and I never understood all the hard plays. This year, some things seem easier. I can run better and don't lose my balance as much. I can kick and hit balls easier, but when I have to run over to one coming in my direction, I get a lot of air. I think the ball is right there, then swoosh, I completely miss it! I know I am getting better, but I still get yelled at sometimes. I just need to get the hang of all these different sports.

Watching your child progress with more understanding of the process makes the entire experience more enriched and ful-filling. Well, hang on—you are just getting

started! There are many more knowledge nuggets up ahead. Kids
who have had some experience with basic play really start to make
bigger gains and learn more skills in the 6- to 9-year-old age group.
By this time, most youngsters have acquired the majority of the basic
fundamental skills to begin more organized sports and exercise
activities. It is an exciting time for children and parents because
everyone can see improvements. Feeling a sense of accomplishment
is one of life's great encouragements and successes. Mastering simple
skills that were previously difficult yields smiles from ear to ear. Just
as an infant can be completely occupied for hours with a plastic ring,
an older child can become ecstatic and overjoyed by acts as simple as
catching or hitting a ball for the first time! We adults need to
remember to always praise and support such achievements, even if
we think they are of minor significance. Things we adults may think
of for a split second may happily occupy a child's mind for days or
weeks. For example, how many weeks do your kids ask you for certain gifts they want for Christmas?

Motor Activity

During the rapid changes experienced by this age group, organization of how the brain talks to the body begins to improve, with
nerve connections doing a better job of communicating the brain's
messages to the muscles to carry out a certain movement. Over time,
that process becomes perfected so movements are more precise.
Throughout this time frame, then, a basic fundamental skill such as
throwing can progress to a transitional skill, such as throwing more
accurately to a specific location.

INSTANT REPLAY

In the 6- to 9-year-old age group, basic fundamental skills can progress to transitional skills.

Running progresses to running more specific patterns with more purpose. Dance movements look more like dance. Transitional skills are critically necessary for graduation to more organized sports activities. Posture, balance, and running usually mature rapidly to adult patterns by about ages 7 to 8 in the majority of children. This concept is very important to understand. Even though children can run, the act of running is not easy for them at first and takes a few years to become a more natural part of their activities without thinking of it as a separate task. This has obvious implications for exercise and sports because running is a skill that is perfected over time just like other skills. We have all seen the difference between running that is painful to watch and running that is smooth and controlled.

Another surprise is that balance control does not come naturally in childhood and requires effort and concentration. Once balance and control of posture mature at around 7 to 8 years of age and become less difficult, certain sports can truly progress. We adults have not had to think about controlling balance and posture because they are so ingrained in our everyday lives. Don't forget that you had to master the ability to maintain balance at some point in your life and that your child needs time to do the same thing and grow into certain abilities. As these functions become automatic, more attention can be directed toward mastering other skills like directional kicking, throwing, catching, aiming for the basket, passing and hitting more precisely for all of the ball sports, better skating patterns, new wrestling or martial arts moves, improved swimming starts, more control of diving and gymnastic stunts, better posture for sports technique, and more specific running patterns. We all wish we could speed up the gears in motion, but doing so is not possible in many cases. Patience will pay off in the long run, allowing your child maximal development of sports skills with minimal pressure.

INSTANT REPLAY

Have the patience to allow your child maximal development of sports skills with minimal pressure.

Visual Ability

The ankle bone may be connected to the knee bone, and the knee bone connected to the hip bone, but the eyeball is not yet completely wired to the brain. By this 6- to 9-year-old age group, the eye has usually achieved its normal round shape and the muscles of the eye can now help track and follow moving objects much better. However, when the signals from the eye get to Grand Central Station in the brain, all the different parts of movement are still difficult to interpret. What this means is that youngsters may be able to judge how fast a ball is moving, but not be able to judge its direction very well, so they will be better with catching, hitting, passing, or kicking a ball that is thrown, hit, passed, or kicked directly to them. Having to figure out where the ball is going and how fast to move to get there is often still difficult. Other sports that don't typically involve flying objects or hand-eye coordination will also show more improvement because of their various and different requirements. For instance, judging walls for flip turns in swimming becomes more easily accomplished because velocity of an approaching wall that is dead center will be easier to process. Now don't go crazy trying to figure out ways to do eyeball exercises to speed up the process—it won't work. There are no eyeball workout videos. Even the Shopping Channel and eBay won't have them. The maturation of visual skills is a natural developmental process that has to happen over time. Remember what your mother always taught you—a watched pot never boils.

Mental Capacity

Attention spans of 6- to 9-year-olds are still short (no joke), and there is difficulty trying to process information from many sources. Most of these children still need a more in-depth form of show-and-tell for instruction. Do not expect them to remember long, detailed directions and carry them out completely, or you risk an episode of brain overload. Unrealistic expectations from instructors can lead to unpleasant situations if children are not able to complete a laundry list of plays. Visual and verbal teaching in short segments is a much more successful approach. Instructors and children feel a sense of accomplishment when many small tasks are completed successfully rather than partially completing a large, complicated task. Remember, some of us are still memory-challenged as adults and can't even remember a grocery list without writing it down. Thank goodness for little sticky notes.

Sports and activities with complex skills require quick assessment of a situation, rapid decision making, and mature levels of transitional skills. Examples of a few of these sports are the more advanced forms of soccer, basketball, hockey, volleyball, baseball, water polo, softball, lacrosse, and football. By all means, kids can be learning the basics of these sports at young ages, but do not expect high levels of performance in most kids in this age group because the development of their memory and complex thinking patterns is still limited. As usual, there are exceptions to every rule. I know some of them personally. If your child is one of those rare cases, celebrate the fact that he is ahead of schedule, let his talent age for a while like a good wine, and be careful not to feel the need for speed or to rush him quickly forward. In general, these activities are hard to grasp beyond the basics for most young children, and the focus should be on continuing to refine basic and transitional skills, general fitness, and technique.

Previously I mentioned that practicing skills among toddlers does not seem to help them improve their ability later on. In contrast, there is evidence to suggest that in the 6- to 9-year-old age group, practicing some skills can produce a more positive effect on overall sports improvement, as well as an advantage of ability when compared with kids who do not practice and then attempt the same skills. This information does not apply to every sport and the research is limited, yet it is encouraging that practicing basic skills at this age can be worth the effort. Don't blow this out of proportion and start over-practicing your child because practicing at this age seems to only benefit a few sports, not all.

Application

In this age group, focus efforts on learning new skills, refining technique, and moving on to transitional skills necessary for eventual increased training and competition. Exposure to a variety of sports activities is highly encouraged. It is a fun time to be coaching, parenting, teaching, and learning, so no emphasis should be put on actual winning. Competition should still be user-friendly with goals being teamwork, improving skills, accomplishing new ones, and making the whole experience a positive one without emphasizing the actual competition. This approach will provide opportunities to applaud for the reality success of your particular child. Children will automatically understand who had more points at the end whether someone talks about winning or losing. Understanding and dealing with wins and losses can be healthy to prepare children for future competition, for events later in life, to focus on the importance of effort, and to see how to improve for the next time. However, these youngsters need to know that the purpose of the practice or event is not who wins, but about outdoing themselves for personal improvement—a big difference. Reality success is thus achieving and accomplishing more things than last time, not necessarily more than somebody else. Swimming, running, tennis, martial arts, skating, volleyball, gymnastics, soccer, basic basketball and hockey, youth league football, and baseball continue to be good suggested choices for elementary schoolchildren, just to name a few.

INSTANT REPLAY

Exposure to a variety of sports activities is highly encouraged.

Reality success is achieving and accomplishing more things than last time, not necessarily more than somebody else.

Having exposure to many different sports activities during this time is important because it allows your child to learn various skills and discover which ones he enjoys doing the most. In general, encouraging exposure to many different sports is very important. Some kids want to try certain sports just because they are cool or the "in" sport at school. That's OK. They will eventually see which activities they like and at which sports they feel they are the most successful.

So, say your child still wants to try football. Believe it or not, some youth football programs have taken parental concerns into consideration and have formed youth leagues that are matched by age, size, and physical maturity. Remember the advantage of T-ball? This is just another example of how to create a positive sports experience by making adjustments for the developmental stage of your active child. Actually, more injuries often occur doing school recess or on jungle gyms, while lower injury rates have been seen in some studies involving youth football because of the adaptations to the general rules that help reduce the potential for injury. If Jermaine plays against Joey because they are roughly the same size, that situation is certainly more equal and fair than playing against someone twice his size. Also, it is important to remember that at younger ages, children do not usually have the strength or speed to generate forces great enough to cause the severe injuries that are seen during adolescence and early adulthood. Injuries rise with advancing age, weight, and level of competition. When parents ask, "When should my child start playing contact sports?" I will spice things up a bit and suggest that it may be more appropriate to ask, "When should my child *stop* playing contact sports?" It's something to think about.

By now, I hope you can see the general ideas, patterns, and themes starting to develop as I travel with you on this incredible yellow brick road called *development*. Most children go through sports skill milestones in a sequence that we cannot change or speed up to the degree most of us would want. However, knowing the way things progress will allow parents, coaches, and doctors to encourage new accomplishments, celebrate little successes, be excited about the ones to come, and not expect a skill way before its time.

INSTANT REPLAY

Most children go through sports skill milestones in a sequence that we cannot change or speed up to the degree most of us would want, so don't expect a skill way before its time.

Sports skill development is a journey, one during which I find many parents and coaches becoming backseat children. "Are we there yet? How many more miles?" Yes, there will be steep uphill grades. Bumps and dips in the road. Dangerous curves ahead. Yet the best part will be the many times you can pull over to appreciate the scenic views. Savor them all.

★ ★ ★ ★ ★ ★ ★ ★ ★ ★ ★ ★ ★ ★ ★ ★ ★

SUCCESS RX

1. Children start to make noticeable gains and learn more skills during the 6- to 9-year-old age group.

2. Basic fundamental skills progress to more transitional skills, while posture, balance, and running mature to more adult patterns by about ages 7 to 8.

3. The eyes can track and follow moving objects much better, but can't judge direction very well.

4. Children have difficulty trying to process information from many sources and also require short instructions. Memory and complex thinking patterns are limited.

5. In this age group, focus efforts on learning new skills, refining technique, and moving on to transitional skills necessary for eventual competition and better performance.

6. Young children need to know that the purpose of the practice or event is not winning, but personal reality success.

7. Exposure to many different sports activities is important because it allows your child to learn various skills and discover which ones he or she enjoys doing the most.

★ ★ ★ ★ ★ ★ ★ ★ ★ ★ ★ ★ ★ ★ ★ ★ ★

Between You and Me

1. Many adults want their children to do a certain sport because it is the one they used to do or know more about. Remember, your child is a wonderful *part* of you, but is *not* you, and may have different interests or attractions, enjoy other sports, or want to become a musical or performing arts athlete. Are you letting your child try many different activities and have a broad base of exposure so he or she can choose what he or she really likes and what produces a sense of accomplishment?

2. Every child has a different rate of growth and development. Can you see roughly where your child is on the long and curvy developmental highway? Are you finding that there are areas that are fast with little traffic, while other areas are bogged down by road construction?

3. It's human nature—we all want to see the finished product and bypass the long process in the middle. Can you imagine how easily adults can get impatient with that developmental process? How do you plan to handle the pressure to push your kid when he or she may not be ready to acquire certain skills?

DNA on Caffeine

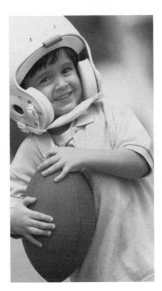

Contact sports are great this year, but I know next year I probably won't play. I am lucky to be on a team where all of us are about the same size, but in the next couple years, no way. Then I will have to play against kids my age who are twice as big as me. I just wish I could grow! I am already 12. What is taking so long? I have good stamina, so maybe I can try running track or swimming.

All of my friends are wondering if they are going to grow. Julie is also 12, but when she came back from summer vacation, I didn't recognizer her! She said she grew so much that she is having trouble practicing her sports, but she is still better than a lot of her teammates. I don't get it.

Gains and achievements in sports skills during the late childhood years continue to happen by leaps and bounds. By the time youngsters reach ages 10 to 12 years, most of them have become good at many different skills—some better than others—and are probably enjoying a few different sports they have realized are fun. Some children may be blossoming in a certain sport. Some may be just beginning to learn a new activity. Some may be enjoying trying them all. It is also a time of rapid flux and dynamic change as children approach and enter puberty at different times. To make things even crazier, girls usually enter puberty before boys. This can be tough in sports in which boys and girls train together, such as running and swimming, because the "already had a growth spurt" girls may start to outperform the "still waiting to have a growth spurt" boys. It's a time when young, budding athletes are finally getting a grip on many skills and seeing progress; when all of a sudden, they are growing 5 inches and tripping over their own shadows. Or they are getting frustrated about standing still while their friends become bigger, stronger, and faster, leaving them in the dust. Learning how to understand and compensate and adjust for growth spurts in your child or her friends can be critical to experience successes during an awkward time when new events throw a pebble in the engine.

INSTANT REPLAY

Learning how to understand and compensate and adjust for growth spurts in your child can be critical to experience successes during an awkward time.

Sometimes this period can make you dizzy, but hang in there. Encouragement and patience can help you and your child weather this developmental tornado and continue to form a positive and lasting impression about exercise and sports. I divided this chapter into 2 sections—the period leading up to puberty (preadolescence) and the period during puberty (adolescence).

Preadolescence

Up to this time, hopefully you have been watching your child's involvement in her activities. Do you get any sense of your child's level of interest or which activity she is enjoying the most? Some preteens may be participating just to exercise and lose weight. Some may enjoy just being involved with their friends. Some may be genuinely interested or talented and want to spend more time learning how to improve at their sport. Whatever the situation, try to figure out which way your child is leaning, and find ways to support the effort. We all see adults around us who are guilty of trying to push, press, and impress that young mind toward a certain sport because that is the sport the adults think is the right choice. Be careful. Kids will gravitate to those activities that are fun for them and give them that feeling of confidence they need to continue in that activity.

INSTANT REPLAY

Kids will gravitate to those activities that are fun for them and give them that feeling of confidence they need to continue.

Remember, we are talking about having reality success in their experiences—which does not depend on the colors gold, silver, or bronze. Some youth enjoy activities or sports, yet may have interests outside of sports as well. That child of yours may share your genes, but she is not a mini-you. Kids are unique with their own set of talents, abilities, likes, and dislikes. And just in case you didn't already know that, just wait until your child becomes a teenager—then she will tell you.

Motor Activity

Preteens have reached a level of development that allows them to really move beyond the fundamental skills and spend more energy fine-tuning transitional and more complex skills. Throwing becomes more accurate. Catching becomes more successful. Passes, shots, and serves are more directed. Motions become more automatic, and actions are much more purposeful in general. Posture and body control continue to improve, making it easier to focus on learning other skills that require good motion control such as turning, pivoting, spinning, and jumping. As skills become more automatic, young athletes can devote more thought and effort to improving the advanced skills required for more significant training and competition.

Visual Ability

Maturation of the eyeball-to-brain pathways improves rapidly to enable more complex patterns of action. Now the brain can see an object, judge where and how fast it is going, and tell the body what to do to get there at the same time. Isn't it amazing how the body works? That ability did not occur because Johnny ate more Wheaties, had a personal trainer, or practiced 4 hours a day starting at age 2. Changes like that happen on a genetic time clock ticking away in the

DNA coupled with good exposure to the sport. Improvement in visual precision has an obvious effect for every sport. Being able to see the swimmer in the next lane while judging the distance to the wall can make all the difference in executing the best possible finish. Seeing where to place the tennis ball, volleyball, or basketball can lead to an ace serve or a made free throw. Visual maturity will help wrestlers and martial artists carry out more difficult moves as their peripheral vision becomes more effective. The implications of visual maturity are obvious for all of the ball sports, as well as sports like diving, gymnastics, and skating that rely on visual markers to perform certain maneuvers.

Mental Capacity

During the preteen years, the brain's ability to plan a set of plays or course of action and store that plan is at a level that allows youngsters to improve in all sports, most notably in those with more complex skills and rapid decision making. These active youngsters should be able to take information input from multiple sources and process it to produce a certain desired action. They can ignore information that is not needed, focus on specific tasks, and make more appropriate decisions with the information they have been given. They become a little less concrete or black-and-white in their thinking patterns and can form a few conceptual thoughts to help build on coaching instructions from the previous months or years. Preteens are able to respond better to verbal instructions with less show-and-tell, but we all know that at any level of sport, visual instruction and demonstration can be worth a thousand words.

Selective attention is improved with less interference from distractions. Pause here for clarification…the key word is *selective*. Johnny may have selective attention on the field to help him perform better, yet also have selective attention and stay focused on the television when asked to take out the garbage.

By this point in development, youngsters should be able to enter basically any sport for more significant competition if they are ready from a mental and emotional standpoint. Don't forget that physical stature is not the only ingredient necessary for successful overall participation. Their bodies may be ready for harder training and competition, but emotionally they need to *know already* that they are valued as your children, regardless of whether they are national, local, or backyard superstars.

Adolescence

So your child has navigated through preadolescence. What comes next? You guessed it…(music from *Jaws* here)…*the teenage years!* Did some of you parents just faint? Relax, if you can. It is an exciting time for most kids involved in sports. The peak of learning sports skills develops during the preteen and teenage years and continues through early adulthood and beyond. Even many adults who were active as teenagers are realizing that they can still perfect their skills, add new ones, and perform sports at very high levels. Yet, the preadolescent and adolescent years encompass the most blurring acceleration of developing and refining sports skills, physical and chemical maturation, and emotional growth. There is also the added bonus of being able to enhance areas of expertise with more devoted training. So hang on to your hats.

Even though there are vast skill improvements during this fast-paced period of adolescence, there are many other important changes that occur during the teen years—and if you blink, you might miss them. The bulk of the topics we should talk about concerning adolescence can be summed up by this P soup—puberty, pounds, plates, performance, and psyche. Puberty, as we all know, can be a wonderful time of growth, maturation, acceptance, achievement, and early independence. It can also be hell on earth for some. Approaching adolescence with a positive attitude can allow your child to see all the changes as a normal and positive part of life.

What is puberty? Growth gone turbo. Garfield becomes Cheetah. Genetics meets Mountain Dew. Besides infancy, adolescence is the only other time in life that you can actually see your kids grow before your very eyes. The changes going on inside that body will blow your mind if it already hasn't. Puberty is the time when youth have their growth spurt, or the most rapid phase of growth. In general, this growth blue-light special usually arrives in girls between ages 11 and 13 and in boys between ages 13 and 15. As we all know, these are just the *average* ages of rapid growth. There are kids all over the map when it comes to the timing of when their body enters puberty. Let me define a couple terms here. Chronological age is defined as your literal age since you were born. Bone age is how old your bones are compared with the average population at a particular stage of bone maturation. Julie can be 13 years old, but have the bones of a 10-year-old because she has not yet gone through puberty. Depending on many factors, children go through puberty at various times. It would be easy if every child hit puberty at the same age, but we did not write those rules.

For example, at 14 years, a normal population of boys can vary by as much as 100 pounds in weight and 5 years in bone age. If this does not give you a scary visual picture, let's pull out a vision chart. I know that you know that I know what I am talking about. Your high-voiced son, who is still 3 years away from a growth spurt, is playing against the man-boy whose baby gift was an electric shaver. Not only would this be a potential setup for injury from a David-and-Goliath scenario, but your child's skeleton is also vulnerable.

Before puberty, the ends of our bones have plates of cartilage that are the areas responsible for making the bones grow longer. These growth plates are unique to kids and consist of layers of growing cartilage sandwiched between bone on either side. Once puberty is over, the growth plate closes and turns to bone. The bone stops growing, and you don't have to buy new clothes for a while—at least until the next fashion trend. However, during childhood and puberty, the surrounding bone, as well as the muscles and tendons, are actually stronger than the soft cartilage growth plate, making it a sitting duck for injury. A sprained ankle in a young growing athlete is less likely to be a ligament sprain and more likely to be an injury to the growth plate because it is the weak link in the bone. Think of the growth plate as an Oreo cookie. It can come apart at its fault line without much force.

Performance can be significantly affected by puberty in positive and negative ways. Increases in body size, hormones, and muscle strength all serve to potentially enhance performance. However, during the period of most rapid growth, there may be a temporary decline in balance skills and body control. With quick increases in height and weight, the body's center of gravity is changed dramatically. New signals from a higher observation point also require adjustments in the brain's interpretation of those signals, and the adolescent may show signs of the "clumsy teenager."

INSTANT REPLAY

During the period of most rapid growth, there may be a temporary decline in balance skills and body control.

Understanding these changes helps prevent a negative reaction to a *normal* developmental process.

This phase can interfere with further progression of skills until the body has adjusted and be especially noticeable in sports that require good balance and body control such as figure skating, diving, gymnastics, and basketball. Don't overlook the fact that longer arms and legs can affect throwing any type of ball, hitting with a bat or racquet, catching with a glove or lacrosse stick, swimming strokes, and jumping hurdles. The key point to remember is that this is a temporary stage of development. Key word—*temporary.* Repeat. Temporary. Did you get it?

Parents have had mental meltdowns when their basketball prodigy grows 8 inches in one year and starts stumbling over his own feet. Parents, coaches, and athletes who understand this process, know it is temporary, and show or receive lots of support enable the young athlete to come out on the other side with a successful result. The goal in this situation is to help prevent a negative reaction to a normal developmental process! Face it—if your child has talent before puberty, that talent should not disappear with a change in stature.

Application

Youth who are successful at early ages are often the ones who enter puberty earlier than their friends. They gain confidence early as they are able to outperform other youth on a regular basis. If possible, these young athletes should be given opportunities to be challenged and train or compete with others of the same maturity level. They should remember that many of their physical advantages will eventually disappear as their peers grow and catch up. In the haste of quick growth and easy sports success, many of these adolescents do not spend the necessary time continuing to perfect their skills. Big mistake! It is still important to concentrate on perfecting the skills of the sport or activity. If your teenager performs better with unrefined raw skills simply because she is bigger and stronger than the other players, she may be unpleasantly surprised when peers catch up and perform better because they have attained a higher skill level.

One of the most dangerous aspects for early maturing children is when their winning ways become *expected.* Coaches and parents become excited about a child's abilities, but the pressure gets turned up when everyone else catches up, becomes the same size, and winning is no longer easy. This pressure can be turned up so much that it causes the child to overtrain and become injured or emotionally shut down and lose heart completely. Hence, the high school star who never produces during college sports or quits because of burnout. Finding opportunities to have your athlete compete or at least train with those who are similarly developed may help lessen these pressurized risks.

If your child's growth spurt is not early or just right, it is late. Late bloomers or late maturers fall into 3 categories—small, overweight, and tall. Late bloomers who are small need guidance about changes to expect as they start to mature and grow. In the meantime, one of the ways to prevent unrealistic expectations is by directing them to sports that are not as dependent on physical size, such as swimming, tennis, martial arts, running, diving, soccer, and gymnastics. Late-maturing kids who are largely overweight may appear perfect to fill the football linebacker position or girl's heavyweight wrestling spot, but their late maturity increases their risk of injury. Even with all that size, they still have bones with immature growth plates and less strength to protect themselves from the opponents of the same size who have already gone through puberty. Late bloomers who are tall may be recruited for the volleyball or basketball team, but until they reach puberty, they may not have the strength or endurance of their peers. The "clumsy teenager" phase may also affect their performance while their teammates have already passed through that stage. Your child should not be held at fault. These circumstances can often be hard for active youngsters to understand, especially if adult figures do not offer correct knowledge, information, or positive support. Knowing what is happening is the first stage of avoiding a potential crisis.

It should be clear now that the physical aspects of youth play a strong role in their ability to participate in sports and exercise. Adolescents are going through such phenomenal changes, self-comparison, and identity investigation that sports do not need to be another straw on the camel's back. Please do not get hung up on developmental deficiencies you can do nothing about. This is not the Da Vinci code. There is no secret to crack. Just understand the process. Understand the stages. Cheer their smallest success. Cheer their best effort. Support them doing exercise. Support them doing sports. Support their athletic and nonathletic endeavors. Support them as your children—period.

★ ★ ★ ★ ★ ★ ★ ★ ★ ★ ★ ★ ★ ★ ★ ★ ★

SUCCESS RX

1. Preteen youth move beyond the fundamentals and can fine-tune transitional and more complex skills. Young athletes can devote more thought and effort to perfect the advanced skills required for more significant training and competition.

2. Maturation of vision pathways improves rapidly to enable more complex patterns of action, including better tracking of moving objects.

3. Preteens should be able to take information input from multiple sources, use more complex thought patterns, and improve rapid decision making.

4. Their bodies may be ready for more intense training and competition, but emotionally they need to already know they are valued as children no matter their achievement level.

5. Puberty usually arrives in girls between ages 11 to 13 and in boys between ages 13 to 15—these ages are just the *average* arrival time for the rapid growth of puberty.

6. If your child matures early, he or she may have a performance advantage over other friends. A dangerous trap to avoid for the early maturing children is when their winning ways become *expected.*

7. During the rapid growth of adolescence and the teen years, there may be a temporary decline in balance and body control as the body's center of gravity is changed and limbs become longer. Remember this fact to help prevent a negative reaction to a *normal* developmental process.

8. Encouragement and patience can help you and your child weather the developmental tornado of adolescence and continue to form a positive and lasting impression of exercise and sports.

★ ★ ★ ★ ★ ★ ★ ★ ★ ★ ★ ★ ★ ★ ★ ★

Between You and Me

1. Sometimes you have some warning when puberty will start if your other children have already experienced it. If this is your first or only child and the average ages for puberty for girls is 11 to 13 years and for boys is 13 to 15 years, do you get a sense that your teenager is developing early or late?

2. Even though your child may be more accomplished at a certain activity, he or she can still acquire important skills from other sports. What can you do to encourage your child to try many different sports?

3. Maybe your child has gravitated to one sport activity. If your child is already specializing in one sport, what can you do to make it a positive, low-pressure experience?

4. Rapid growth can affect many skills and abilities as the body changes dramatically. Do you view this as a threat to your child's talent, or can you support your athlete through this temporary stage?

Cellular Success

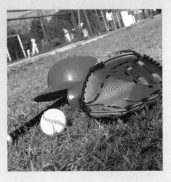

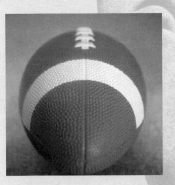

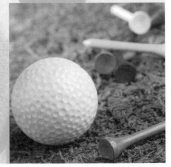

Body Chemistry

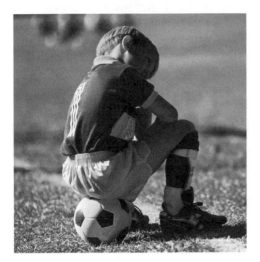

*W*hew! Running is fun, but I just can't seem to get a lot faster! I don't know why. I am running more than I was the past 2 years put together. I keep hearing, "You have to run more distance to improve your running times," so I keep trying. I have run more and I even got some great new shoes, but I just make small improvements in my times. How come I run more than Joey and he keeps getting faster all the time?

Refining and perfecting motor skills, developing visual precision, and improving mental sharpness are just a few of the many achievements happening in the young, growing body that contribute significantly to your youngster's enjoyable and successful reality sports experience. Think about shaking up a soft drink can and not opening the top—there is so much rapid change just waiting to happen in these kids. Sometimes they can sense that they are close to gaining a new skill and they just about burst trying. Suddenly it happens, and they cheer not only with excitement, but relief. Hopefully you can see that each stage of development varies in the length of time it takes to gain accomplishment with a certain skill and also in the completeness of skills actually developed. Some youth will acquire a skill fairly quickly, while others take longer. Some youth will develop a certain skill very well, while others struggle. That's why certain kids gravitate toward certain activities—the beauty of the variability of human beings.

Think back to your childhood for a moment. Did you excel at catching and hitting baseballs, or were you hand-eye challenged and avoided that type of activity altogether? Did you throw well, or did you hate dodgeball in PE class when you had to display your lack of ability in front of the whole class? Ah, now you remember. You may see that mirror image in your child, or you may be wondering how on earth he inherited abilities you do not have.

Even with this variability among children of skills for exercise and sports, it is important to allow each child to individually maximize each skill level in his own time before moving on to the next. Each child is unique and should not be pushed faster than the time required to refine a skill needed to acquire a future skill. This book is about allowing your child to achieve the most personal improvement and achievement. The most accomplishment. The most potential. The best experience in his athletic endeavors. Remember not to become impatient and rob your young one of the chance to gain a particular skill that he has been working on so diligently. Sure, your child can occasionally be trying more advanced parts of a sport, but he should not be rushed to get there before the current skills are mastered. When we were kids in school, next year's classes were usually built on knowledge from the previous year. Taking calculus before algebra and geometry would not have made as much sense (although for a non–math wizard like me, I am not sure if calculus would have made sense at any time). It is the same with acquiring the different advancing levels of sports techniques, movements, strategies, and training. One step at a time. One throw at a time. One serve at a time. One jump at a time. One kick at a time.

Motor, visual, and mental skills, along with physical growth, only make up part of the overall picture. They are each contributing parts that all fit together. Have you ever searched for that missing piece that allows you to start to assemble the next large chunk of a complicated puzzle? Advancing maturation of the body and brain allow your child to benefit from advancing physical growth. Sure, these physical changes of growth are obvious. No one is blind to the fact that when friends get your holiday picture this year, Johnny is 6 inches taller than last year's picture (which is still on their refrigerator). They usually double-check to make sure you did not skip a year. Girls change shape and start looking at boys; boys start to shave, get more muscles, and look at girls. These physical changes certainly have an effect on their abilities to perform against their opponents as they become stronger, faster, and more skilled. Just growing, however, is not the only answer in the game of sports Jeopardy. We have previously discussed how motor skills develop in a sequence that allows kids to gradually acquire abilities; physical growth enhances the use of those new abilities. Yet the iceberg is still partially underwater. Another crucial factor that goes through a process of development is the more invisible chemical realm—*physiology,* in fancy medical terms.

INSTANT REPLAY

Another crucial area that goes through a developmental process is the more invisible chemical realm of *physiology.*

The contributions from the body's chemical makeup can be just as important to a youngster's ability to have a great sports experience as the contributions from vision and coordination that let Johnny progress from T-ball to baseball, or Julie progress from forehands to backhands, or Jermaine progress from free throws to three-pointers. Understanding these processes can continue to enhance the sports experience for everyone involved, especially your child. This under-standing can reduce adult pressures to perform or train beyond what the young body can master. During the winding course of sports development, motor skills may be developed, but the physiology may not. "Gee," you say, "this is more complex than I thought!" It is amazing how many problems of pressure can be caused simply by a lack of knowledge and understanding about the tremendous devel-opmental changes that occur in your child. There is a lot to know and understand about how your child can have a positive encounter with sports and exercise without being overloaded. I know it is a lot of information and may even be a bit overwhelming at times. Just

like in school, it will be worth knowing. And don't worry, the only
test at the end of this book is not on paper, but in everyday life with
your child.

As with other skill development, these chemical properties are
influenced by genetics, develop in a progressive manner, and primarily
improve with training when the timing is right. Consider Superman
when he was a child. What do we know about little Clark Kent's childhood? When he was finally given his first cape with a small letter "s"
on the front, I doubt if he was immediately able to fly and leap tall
buildings. He was still taking baby leaps. His cape size had to be
changed as he grew, and I am sure it had to be mended a few times.
Then he had to learn the best ways to use his abilities over time.
Not until he went through puberty and changed from Superboy
to Superman was he able to maximize his powers. He didn't just
step into his cape—he grew into it. Some of your children will have
invisible capes and experience a lot of winning ways in their sports
activities. Others will have no cape, yet still achieve a lot of personal
accomplishment in their sports activities. Both are reality. Both are
successful. Both are Superkids.

Sports and exercise performance is influenced by many things
outside and within the body. Outside (external) factors that play a
role in sports performance include equipment, coaching, finances,
and available opportunity. Most equipment issues are fairly equal
among youngsters because everyone usually has the same general
type of gear. Coaching styles can differ significantly, but a style
that works well for one child may not work at all for another. Some
sports are more costly in which to participate, making it difficult for

some children to ever find out if that is where their talent was. Even our local environments can make it challenging for all children to be exposed to different sports and exercise opportunities, whether because of weather issues or safety concerns. Despite the effect outside factors have on the way your child develops in sports, our inside (internal) factors also have a profound effect on sports performance. Many of these internal factors are part of the chemical or physiologic aspect of the body. As with motor development, there are physiologic skills that develop progressively. They develop alongside motor skills, yet at a different pace and time sequence, and are just more ingredients in the bigger pie of skill development.

INSTANT REPLAY

Sports performance and ability are influenced by many things outside and within the body.

Application

Maturation of the chemical processes in the body will enable your youngster to enhance the motor skills that he is mastering as he grows. Some of these chemical insiders of physiology include aerobic capacity and training ability, body composition and flexibility, growth, and heat tolerance. You can see how these all go hand in hand with motor skills and add to the wide range of abilities among children. Any type of sport or recreational activity will be affected by how aerobic development affects speed and endurance, flexibility affects form and technique, and heat tolerance affects exercise, training, and performance. Strength also contributes significantly to bursts of power or long, repetitive activities, but that topic gets a whole chapter to itself later on. Stay tuned.

★ ★ ★ ★ ★ ★ ★ ★ ★ ★ ★ ★ ★ ★ ★ ★ ★

SUCCESS RX

1. Despite a lot of variability from child to child, it is important to allow each child to individually maximize each skill level in his or her own time before moving on to the next.

2. Motor, visual, and intellectual development plus physical growth contribute to part of the entire picture of a youngster's abilities. Another crucial developmental factor involves body chemistry, also known as *physiology*.

3. Understanding these processes can help enhance the experiences of various exercise and sports involvement.

4. Chemical development progresses in a pace and sequence that occurs alongside physical development.

★ ★ ★ ★ ★ ★ ★ ★ ★ ★ ★ ★ ★ ★ ★ ★ ★

Between You and Me

1. Continue to support the development of skills you can visibly see. The unseen chemical development will show itself in different ways. Have you noticed how your child may be different than other kids when it comes to flexibility or the ability to run longer?

2. Remember that development of all facets is still development and doesn't happen overnight. Try not to rush ahead or predict certain abilities. What abilities does your child have that you can applaud right now?

The Invisible Factory

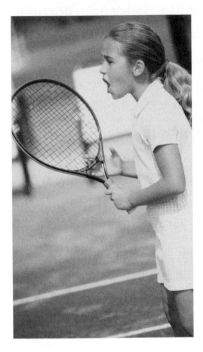

Oh my gosh! I can't believe it! I am finally having more speed and endurance. Last year, I was always slower than my friends. Jose was faster in soccer, Jalial was faster in track, Jodie was faster in swimming, and Ju-Lin always outlasted me in tennis. It just wasn't cool because I worked so hard in PE class and in all the sports I like. But now, I am working just as hard and it seems to be making a difference. I can go faster and last longer. It may not make sense, but I sure like it!

Chemical actions are happening in your body all the time, just like a busy factory, and even continue to happen in your sleep. You and your child may not always feel these actions or be able to see them, but the tiny cells in your body rely on these chemical processes to keep them alive and functioning. This chemical part of your child—the physiology—is necessary for many aspects of sports participation and improving or enhancing certain motor skills. The chemical nature of muscles is what helps determine whether your child will be better at strength and power activities or better able to excel in endurance sports or highly repetitive activities. The chemical ability to use oxygen in the body can affect how long your child can sustain high levels of activity. The chemical structure of tissues will enable your child to have more flexibility. The chemical nature of a young child affects responses to the environment, and the chemical changes with puberty affect many things like strength, growth, endurance, and adjusting to the local climate. It's exciting to see how the physical changes work with the chemical to continue to enhance and optimize your child's overall development for exercise activities and sports of all kinds. Let's look at a few of these aspects of physiology and how they can apply to your child.

INSTANT REPLAY

Chemical (physiologic) development is necessary for many aspects of sports participation and improving or enhancing certain motor skills to optimize your child's overall sports development.

Aerobic Capacity and Training Ability

Aerobic capacity refers to a child's ability to sustain a certain level of aerobic activity for a certain length of time. An aerobic activity is one that requires oxygen exchange in the blood to a greater degree than other activities, such as running versus strength training. Being able to sustain aerobic activity for longer periods of time depends on the body's ability to transport oxygen to the tissues and muscles of the body and then use it efficiently once it gets there. In the scientific world, our aerobic capacity can be measured and is called VO_2 *max*. In a broken nutshell, VO_2 max is the maximum level of the body's ability to effectively take up oxygen, transport it, and use it for sustained exercise energy.

Normally, in adults, this ability to use oxygen can be improved with training and exercise. Improvements can be made with as little as 15 to 20 minutes of exercise 3 times a week. If you exercise more, your aerobic capacity can continue to improve to a certain point before it levels off. The interesting point about children is that even when recommendations for adult exercise are used, only small improvements (approximately 5%–10%) in aerobic capacity are seen until your child reaches puberty. Additional improvements can result simply from their ability to do the movements more easily, more efficiently, and with more motivation.

INSTANT REPLAY

Even when using exercise recommendations for adults, only small improvements in aerobic ability are seen until a child reaches puberty.

On the other hand, some youngsters do not show any improvement with the amount of training that often leads to predictable gains in adults. Don't despair! Once your active youngster goes through puberty, aerobic capacity can blossom. So let me reemphasize—training kids as adults does not necessarily lead to adult results and can often lead to adult injuries. Training kids as kids within their bodies' boundaries can lead to their best potential results. Another important concept is that your child may genetically have a better ability for aerobic activity, but she still has to have the motor development and motivation to use it for a positive effect on ability and the sports experience.

INSTANT REPLAY

Training kids as adults does not necessarily lead to adult results and can often lead to adult injuries.

Training kids as kids within their bodies' boundaries can lead to their best potential results.

Acceptable levels of training will accomplish many good results and allow your child to progress nicely when the appropriate levels of development have been reached. I feel you tapping me on my shoulder. Yes, there are kids whose development is so progressed that they can train as adults even when they are young, and I have seen many of them. Think about teenagers in the Olympics, for example. It was very exciting for me to be one of the Olympic doctors and see some teenagers produce stellar performances. I realized that they had been able to train at significant levels even at younger ages because their bodies had matured earlier and were ready to handle such training, and also because of genetic influences. The timing of puberty obviously has a profound effect on gaining aerobic improvement, among other things. Sports readiness such as this will be significantly different among youngsters of the same age. Some will be ready a lot earlier than others because they develop and reach puberty more quickly. In some cases, their motor development is already capable of responding to the early maturation of aerobic development, as was the case with those young Olympians. In other cases, youngsters go through puberty early, but still need their motor skills to catch up with their new and improved aerobic abilities. Each athlete is different. Some improve at an early age; some improve much later. Some improve a lot; some barely improve at all. How far and in what direction these improvements occur still depend on the genetic makeup of your child and where along the genetic spectrum she lies—anywhere from pure strength and power sports, to medium strength and aerobic sports, to very aerobic sports and anywhere in between.

The general concepts still apply—until puberty, there is a limited ability to improve aerobic capacity just by training alone. Once puberty is reached, improvements in your child's ability to use oxygen occur rapidly and progressive gains can be made. Although it appears that there is a certain unseen upper limit to improve aerobic capacity before puberty, this does not reduce or lessen the need to train aerobically. This is a very important distinction. There is strong evidence that young athletes with a good foundational base of aerobic exercise can have even better improvements in aerobic ability once they reach puberty than those who start aerobic training at a later age. For example, a swimmer or runner who has already had some years of moderate training before her growth spurt has a better aerobic base from which to improve once puberty arrives. Kids who train in aerobic sports also better their performance because of improved technique and efficiency of movement, advancing skill level, maturing coordination, and growing motivation. Understanding the place of aerobic development in the bigger picture is important in the younger years to take the focus away from competition, time or speed qualifications, and excessive training schedules. This understanding allows your child to focus instead on having fun, improving technique, learning different sports skills, and developing a strong base level of aerobic conditioning.

Hopefully this is clear. Read my lips—there is *no need* for elaborate, excessive, and exhaustive training programs for children and prepubertal athletes. This does not suit their needs or interests. Parents, coaches, and kids who are not informed about this process may be the victims of discouragement when children do not get significantly faster as their level of training increases. Unfortunately, in those circumstances, increased training continues to be enforced with the thought that more is better and necessary to get the desired effect. When these training loads increase beyond a certain point, young bodies and minds start to break down. On the other hand, when training is kept at the right level and combined with positive reinforcement, support, emphasis on technique, opportunities for participation, new skill trials, and a focus on having fun, young bodies and minds can develop and accomplish their maximum potential ability more successfully.

INSTANT REPLAY

There is no need for excessive, elaborate, or exhaustive aerobic training programs in children.

Once puberty is reached, improvements in the ability to use oxygen occur rapidly, and progressive gains can be made if there has been a good base of moderate aerobic training.

What's the "right" level of aerobic training, you ask? Every child will be different because of stage of development and chemical makeup. The important thing is to pay attention to your child's development. If puberty has not started to show signs of its debut, maintaining moderate aerobic training loads is adequate. Your athlete can still improve by perfecting technique, consistent training, and maintaining good nutrition. When the chemical bonanza of puberty arrives, then ta-da! At that point, increased aerobic training will have much more potential to add to motor skills and enhance ability if there has been enough patience in you, your child, and the coach to avoid the temptation to over-increase training.

This is an extremely important concept to grasp. Consider the following 2 scenarios. Julie A has more genetic talent for aerobic sports and easily achieves some wins at an early age, but has a coach and parents who feel that the only way for her to get faster is to continue to increase her training load. When her improvements start to level off (as she reaches that upper limit of aerobic ability before puberty), she is pushed harder and subjected to heavier and heavier training loads. She gets hurt with an overuse injury and then loses her desire. Once she reaches puberty, she lacks the motivation to train hard enough to take advantage of her increased physiologic ability. She does not have enough wins to consider herself successful (or to be considered successful by her parents), so she suffers from burnout and eventually quits the sport.

On the other hand, Johnny B has less genetic ability, but is fortunate to be trained by a coach who spends more time refining his technique, building his confidence, and maintaining an adequate conditioning program. His parents encourage him to be patient for puberty while his teammates are growing all around him, and they show great support by showing up to his events and cheering his improvements whether he wins or loses. He concentrates on doing his best and uses his better form and technique to challenge his competitors. When he reaches puberty, he is ready to respond to the aerobic challenge of harder training sessions with dramatic improvements in performance, leading to many years of achievement in his sport. Who had the most talent? Julie A. Who achieved reality success? Correct answer—Johnny B. I know, because that was me.

Body Composition and Flexibility

These 2 areas help remind us that children are different from adults and each other. It may seem ridiculous to speak about body composition and flexibility in kids because we all know they are mostly made of Play-Doh. However, it is important to discuss the general changes in body tissues that occur during growth and the various effects these changes have on exercise and sports participation.

Girls and boys can play together until about the third grade. After this point, it is a good idea to start the transition of separating boys and girls in contact-type sports. This gives plenty of time for puberty to start and not have a 4'2", 70-pound boy playing against a 5'9", 130-pound girl. Remember, the average ages that puberty begins is much different for girls and boys. Even from early childhood, girls in general have more body fat than boys. That is just the way the cards are dealt. Differences in body fat stay throughout childhood and then increase in girls once they hit puberty. Boys have a more dramatic change in body composition because new levels of testosterone from puberty start to add muscle mass. Kids who are already overweight tend to remain overweight into adolescence and adulthood. The changes in body composition are important because they may have an effect on sports participation and performance, especially in sports in which center of gravity and weight are important like gymnastics, diving, figure skating, and wrestling. Puberty is a time of multiple adjustments that can have an effect on your child's participation in sports. Understanding the reality of the physical and chemical changes of puberty can enable you to support your active child during and through that period of development.

Children are also more flexible than adults. Who do you think was the model for Gumby? It had to be a child. But as usual, many good things must come to an end or just slow down. During the rapid growth of puberty, kids often become temporarily less flexible than they were prior to puberty. Let me paint a visual for you here. Some children have a slow growth spurt, while others grow so fast they need a speeding ticket. Essentially, their bones are growing more quickly than their muscles and tendons can stretch to keep up. Most boys get more muscles and lose some body fat, but often lose flexibility. Girls can also become tighter during the rapid growth of puberty if they cannot stretch to keep up with their growth. However, the increase in estrogen usually allows girls to maintain or improve their flexibility once they slow down their speed of growth. Having good flexibility may help some athletes self-select into certain sports such as swimming, diving, gymnastics, tennis, figure skating, wrestling, or martial arts. Understanding these changes in body composition and flexibility can prepare you for their potential effect as you watch your child exercise, train, or compete while going through puberty.

Growth

When observing youngsters who participate in good exercise programs with good nutrition, it is fun to watch their bodies grow and take healthy shapes. Exercise, for the most part, is considered important for promoting growth and development. Rewind. Let me say it once again—exercise is good and an important contributor to overall health. This book is here to support exercise and all the benefits that come along with it. However, in my sports medicine clinic, I see too many kids who are hurt because they are pushed too hard or push themselves too hard because they feel pressured. This type of scenario occurs with athletic youth as well as with those who are overweight; both groups can fall into the same trap. I think we have come a long way from Popeye and his spinach to the "Got Milk?" advertisements, but we may have gone overboard with all the supplements and over-intense exercise programs out there that your kids are being suckered into as the "right thing." How many times did your mother tell you that too much of a good thing was not good? Of course, she was talking about chocolate, but the idea applies here, too. There is a lot of hot debate about whether some sports activities can actually have a negative effect on growth if taken too far.

In some cases, it appears that intense, hard-core, adult-level exercise in kids can hinder their overall growth. It does not appear that the sports themselves are truly bad for growth; it's how exercise can be used in excessive ways that is the culprit. If high levels of exercise are combined with improper nutritional balance, overly restricted caloric intake, and a lack of rest, the body cannot sustain the energy needed to grow properly. This often shows up after athletes stop the sport or have time off because of an injury and then have catch-up growth to that of their peers. The math equation for this is too many calories burned, plus not enough calories taken in (or too many calories restricted), plus a lack of proper recovery time, equals not enough calories to allow the body to grow.

Heavy intense training requires and burns significant calories. Rapid growth of puberty requires significant calories. Heavy intense training at young ages while the body is still growing burns an extraordinary amount of calories. This is not higher math here. How many of you live with human disposals? They graze through the countertops, cabinets, and refrigerator every 30 minutes scouring for food—and still have trouble gaining or maintaining weight. If significant calories are lacking when they are needed to help maintain exercise and growth, growth will lose out and the calories will be used to sustain those high levels of exercise. When this type of restriction is done *intentionally,* it brings to mind small calves growing in confined wooden crates to produce the best veal. On a positive note, most cases are not at all intentional, but just a combination of a talented, athletic youngster who is unable to meet caloric needs and is maintaining a heavy training load while the body is growing rapidly. Nutrition and intense exercise are not the only factors that can affect growth. Some of the youngsters in these sports are already genetically smaller to start with. Growth can also be affected by illness or injury because these conditions also require adequate nutrition to help the body heal.

I am definitely not pointing fingers at any particular sport. I am pointing out very profound points about any strenuous exercise program that you should understand so you can not only protect your child's ability to train and improve, but also protect your child's ability to grow. Aren't these good things? Just like the theme of the rest of this book—I challenge you with these points to assist you in reasoning and understanding ways to help maximize potential, minimize pressure, and obtain the reality success your child deserves. There are areas of concern to which we must pay attention because of what the young body needs during different stages of development. This line of thinking isn't to change certain sports, but to provide discussion to understand the process of growth for you to act appropriately to provide healthy growth and development for your child while being active in any sporting activity.

Heat Tolerance

There have been far too many young athletes who have died from heat stroke or suffered severe heat exhaustion from training in the heat and unfortunately, heat stroke is one of the common causes of exercise-related death in high school students in the United States.

Deadly combinations usually involve high heat and humidity, but similar catastrophic problems have occurred in less drastic climates. Long before your child moves up to high school sports, the issues of heat tolerance need your utmost attention. Compared with adults, children's ability to tolerate the heat is very different. Once again, development is waving its flag, wanting to be seen and heard. If it was visible, it would be jumping up and down saying, "Pick me! Pick me!" This child-adult difference in handling heat is important if you have a child who is training in a sport that is outdoors or traveling to other states to compete, especially in geographic areas where temperature and humidity are known to be high. This difference can certainly affect the way your child is able to train and perform. Knowledge about how your youngster developmentally handles heat can hopefully help prevent serious or even mild problems.

INSTANT REPLAY

Compared with adults, children's ability to tolerate heat is very different.

There are quite a few basic differences in the chemical makeup of children that make it harder for them to regulate body temperature than adults.

1. Children have more body surface area than body weight, so when the outside temperature is higher than body temperature, children tend to gain heat faster than adults. Don't let their smaller size deceive you.

2. During exercise, children generate up to 20% to 25% more heat for their body weight than adults. Youngsters' higher metabolic rates also contribute to the higher amounts of heat that kids can generate with exercise and activities.

3. Movements that are unrefined and inefficient produce more heat in kids than older athletes who have mastered their techniques and have more smooth movements.

4. The amount of blood pumped during exercise is less in children than adults, so there is less ability to move heat to the skin to give off heat.

5. Children have immature sweating mechanisms and also sweat less than adults, so they have less ability to get rid of heat by evaporation of sweat. They do not have as many sweat glands, and those sweat glands are not as efficient as adults. Getting sunburned also decreases the ability of the sweat glands to perform, so wearing sunscreen is a must (in addition to protecting their skin from premature aging and skin cancer).

6. Children adjust to the heat more slowly, so it will take longer for them to get used to summer temperatures and humidity than adults. This process of adaptation is called acclimatization. This ability to adapt is what allows your Baby Bear not to get too hot or too cold, but to be just right.

7. Core body temperature in children rises higher and more quickly with dehydration, so it is even more important to provide drink breaks for young active children. The thirst drive in a child is not as good as an adult's thirst drive, so taking frequent breaks to drink fluids should be mandatory.

8. Children who are overweight are even more at risk for heat illness
   because extra weight can compound most of these problems. They
   have to generate more heat to move the larger body mass,
   it is harder to give off heat (so they retain more heat), and they
   adjust even more slowly to the heat.

Application

Understanding the chemical/physiologic changes that occur during
development adds to the complexity of how your child acquires her
sports skills for activities of all kinds and accomplishes milestones
along the reality path of sports and exercise. Makes you think, doesn't
it? There is a lot more going on than you ever imagined. It isn't just
enough to understand how motor skills come along and improve—
those motor abilities can be affected by chemical development. It is
difficult to completely take advantage of physical or physiologic
talent until both are more fully developed. Everything is very inter-
twined. All aspects are interconnected. Each one is important. Sports
Skills Development 101 is becoming more complex, yet is a definite
prerequisite for Reality Sports Success 201.

★ ★ ★ ★ ★ ★ ★ ★ ★ ★ ★ ★ ★ ★ ★ ★ ★

SUCCESS RX

1. Chemical (physiologic) development affects and enhances your child's ability to use his or her motor skills such as being able to run longer distances as endurance capabilities improve.

2. The timing of puberty has a profound effect on aerobic improvement, so moderate aerobic training programs are adequate prior to puberty.

3. Youngsters with a good foundational base of aerobic training can have better improvements in aerobic ability once they reach puberty.

4. Changes in body composition affect participation because of effects on body weight, flexibility, muscle strength, and body fat.

5. There are important differences in the chemical makeup of children that make it harder for them to adapt to the heat and regulate body temperature than adults.

★ ★ ★ ★ ★ ★ ★ ★ ★ ★ ★ ★ ★ ★ ★ ★ ★

Between You and Me

1. Maybe it is not yet clear where your child falls on the spectrum of aerobic activity. Is your child working on improving technique and skills, or just training more?

2. Suppose you see that your child has an affinity for more endurance-type activities. Try to keep in perspective how puberty affects aerobic ability. Are you able to avoid the temptation to push for higher loads of training before it would be appropriate?

3. Many exciting changes occur physically and chemically that can contribute to a substantial improvement in sports abilities. Are you continuing to cheer achievement, accomplishment, and self-improvement? Are you more mindful now of the different developmental changes so you can be careful not to put unnecessary pressure on your active child?

4. There are many chemical responses that are underdeveloped in your child compared with adults, such as the ability to deal with the heat. Understanding these differences will hopefully help reduce the risks of heat problems and how your child responds to the heat. Are you more aware now to be sure your child is wearing sunscreen and has drinking fluids available at all times?

Mental Success

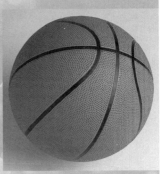

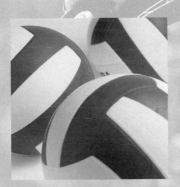

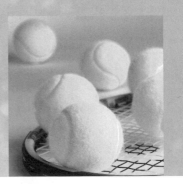

A Firm Foundation

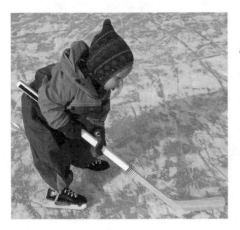

This is sooooo fun! I love getting to play. This coach is great. He lets us change players every 3 plays and everyone gets a high five, no matter how we played. He doesn't even keep score. Last year wasn't like that at all because the coach was more worried about how she looked rather than how we looked, so she would always get mad if we didn't win.

Look at Joey. He still doesn't seem to have a good time. I guess it's because he is always worrying if something is wrong with him if he doesn't score every time. I don't know why he puts so much pressure on himself, but maybe it comes from home. His parents don't show up at very many games, and when they do, they only speak up if he does something wrong. He's definitely the best one on the team, but he is never happy. That's so weird.

I'm glad my folks are here most of the time and they just cheer when I am out there. How funny. But at least I don't have to worry if I mess up. They just tell me to learn from my mistakes, try again, and keep going. This game is hard enough, so when I hear my parents yell, "Good job, Johnny!" I know they mean it.

Just when you thought there could not be more, there is more. It's not enough to understand the developmental milestones of growth and the maturation process of skills for sports activities. Nor is it enough to appreciate the chemical development that affects ability. Yes, all the physical changes, chemical changes, and developmental sequences must be considered and incorporated into the challenges of accomplishment and performance in the youth sports experience. Yet even all of those ingredients do not make up the whole enchilada. There is still more that is necessary to complete the menu—the rice, beans, and salsa. The development of mental (psychological) skills is also incredibly important for these youngsters and completes the third part of the triangle of components that all mesh together to influence the athletic potential of your child. All 3 are of major significance and really cannot function maximally without the other 2 being in place. Your child may be ready for intense competition from a standpoint of muscular control, technique, and skill level, but not from a mental or emotional standpoint. Your child may have successfully mastered how to integrate skills with maturing chemical processes of speed, strength, and endurance, but still be insecure or immature when it comes to advancing levels of performance. If the child is subjected to competition and heavy training before psychological development is ready, the results can be disastrous. If parents, coaches, teachers, and instructors understand these principles and how they can connect the dots, we are definitely on our way to a positive sports experience for everyone involved.

INSTANT REPLAY

The development of mental *(psychological)* skills is incredibly important and completes the third part of the triangle of components that all mesh together to influence the athletic potential of your child.

If you have heard conversations between kids, you know they spend a lot of their time comparing lives. "My dad can leap tall buildings." "My mom drives a faster car." "My video game is harder than yours." "My big brother is bigger than your big brother." "Whatever you can do, I can do better." Youngsters start to develop ideas about themselves by comparing their skills to those of other children and siblings. They also start to add to their self-esteem by interpreting how others respond to their actions. This comparison activity starts as early as around 5 years of age, so you can see how the mental aspect of reality sports success also develops over time just like the other areas we have been discussing. These mental canvases gradually become painted with a picture that forms a substantial artwork foundation and scenic self-image on which your child continues to add colors. Paint can be

added in positive and negative ways. Sometimes, your child inter-
prets reactions from someone else in a completely different way than
the other person intended. Adults must be very careful about the
words they choose. Sarcasm and joking may work with fellow adult
peers, but may be taken personally by a child.

Because formation of self-image starts at a relatively early age, we
adults have some important years to enforce and reinforce positive
value in our youngsters—precious years to start the foundation of a
positive definition of success and accomplishment before any serious
competition gets started. Take advantage of those years! Substantial
formation of self-concepts becomes ingrained early in life, and trying to change that in later years may be very difficult or impossible.
All eyes right here—you will rarely have a better opportunity to positively influence how your kid thinks about himself than when he is
young. If you wait too long, not only are negative concepts difficult
to reverse, but mediocre self-images are difficult to improve because
they have already become ingrained at a certain level of value. We
have all seen it happen—children who have already accepted either
a life of accomplishment or a life of no achievement based on what
they have been told over and over. More positive paint or more
negative paint. A canvas painting fit for one of the best museums
in the world, or one placed on a barren wall that is rarely seen.

INSTANT REPLAY

You will rarely have a better opportunity to positively
influence how your kids think about themselves than
when they are young.

Think about this tremendous opportunity you have. See this occasion as a treat. What a phenomenal opportunity we have as adults to add beautiful paint. I am sure some of you never had that as a child or had horrible pressure placed on you to be a sports star, but I guarantee that you can break the trend and keep it from continuing with your own child. On the flip side, some of you may be a branch on a family tree full of sports superstars, yet have a child who just isn't interested or is afraid of not being able to carry on the family tradition. You have the ability to help encourage what interests your child *does* have or help defuse the bomb of high expectations. Whatever the talents or deficits are, please don't let your child be parentally impaired.

One of many life-changing experiences I've had involved working at a large youth sports camp where we could only speak positively with the kids and encourage them. Always finding something positive to say was difficult to do for some, as you can imagine, but it was sheer joy to see the transformation of these young people in just a month after they realized that they *could* do something right and began seeing themselves more confidently. Hmm...it's amazing to see what happens when people start hearing good things about themselves.

The positive change affected us camp counselors as much as the kids because it became a habit to think and speak positively and always search for what other people were doing well. It took effort to look beyond the rough surface of some of the attitudes. It took a lot of time to listen to the mind that was inside that freckled face. It took unselfishness to spend time with the kids and watch what made them tick. It took swallowing pride to remove our expectations and preconceived ideas to allow the youngster to pursue the things for which he had a desire, and then watch him surprise us with what he had inside. The important thing to remember about this process is that it should be standard practice whether your child is an athlete, is involved in recreational sports, is interested in art or music, or loves to read books. Actions do speak loudly, but words also impact with major volume. Our world is surrounded by so much negativity—the news on television, magazines, newspapers, tabloids, and music. It is easy to just fall into that same habit and run with the lemmings as they jump off a cliff. But you don't have to. You can start pushing that snowball uphill and form a new habit of the way you look at things—especially now that you have greater knowledge of the developmental phenomenon. So many of our actions are the way they are because that is what we learned. I fix it this way because that's the way my dad fixed it. I cook it this way because that's they way my grandmother cooked it. How often do you stop to think about those hand-me-down habits and rituals? They may be great, or there just might be a better way now.

Children have so much to gain from participating in various physical activities. Besides influencing self-esteem, participation can enhance leadership qualities, character development, the concept of teamwork, discipline, and self-confidence because of self-improvement. If the experience is a positive one, it can affect their view of sports and exercise for a lifetime. Athletes who stay involved in activities long term have a definite passion and excitement that keeps them involved even through long hours and years of discipline and sacrifice. An important goal is to make sure the excitement is not replaced by pressure and stress.

We have all seen the excitement children have when opening presents or catching their first ball. Their smiles expand a mile, their bodies shake, and they start bouncing uncontrollably like a Super Ball in a box. Being excited about an activity is a normal response and something we all desire. Another normal response in athletics is the brief stress associated with a performance, including butterflies in the stomach, increased heart rate, and nervousness. Significant stress, on the other hand, involves fear of the event. When a child senses or hears high levels of expectations, he can become fearful of not being able to live up to those expectations. Some interesting points have turned up during scientific research. Stress before an event is often related to how a child thinks he is capable of performing that activity. Stress after an event is usually related to how a child perceives his actual performance. Among children, the most important factor that lowers stress after an event is the amount of fun experienced by the child, whether they were on the winning or losing team.

INSTANT REPLAY

When a child senses or hears high levels of expectations, he or she can become fearful of not being able to live up to those expectations.

But what about that pre-event stress? If it is based on the way a youngster thinks he will perform, it is easy to see how some confidence going into the event could help reduce stress and anxiety, especially if he is not fearful of what will happen if he doesn't achieve that winning level of performance. This is exactly where the youngster's inner definition of reality success makes a big difference. In some cases, young people have lower levels of self-confidence despite positive parental and coaching input. This just means these kids need more praise, which may take a special effort on the part of the adults to find that area of improvement. Parents and coaches who do not require a lot of praise or attention themselves might not give as much or know how to give as much. Yet each child is unique in the amount of praise required to help build self-confidence and self-esteem. Live and learn what your child needs. Your children may be from you and your spouse, but they are all different in their needs. Johnny's confidence can come merely from knowing that he is supported *unconditionally* if he tries his best. Janae can better focus on her skills if she can relax about the outcome. Yes, there are always times for correction of mistakes during sports activities; that is part of the learning process. Although constructive corrective advice from a parent is not wrong, it may be perceived by the child as a negative statement or criticism if it occurs too often. Remember how sometimes your youngster will listen to other people better than you just because they aren't his parent? Each situation is unique, but much of the correction should be left up to the coach or instructor. For instance, if a swimmer has improved his butterfly technique, but still needs work on perfecting the turn at the wall, make sure you praise the improved technique and allow the coach to provide positive feedback and constructively correct the less-than-optimal turns.

Prominent viewpoints circling youth sports are numerous, but the majority of concepts involve

- Decreasing the emphasis on winning
- Increasing the emphasis on having fun

- Giving one's best effort
- Learning sportsmanship
- Gaining better fitness levels
- Improving sports skills

What a novel idea—kids just want to have fun. That may come as a shock to some of you, but it is a normal phenomenon of psychological development for children to be more concerned with the activity than with the outcome.

INSTANT REPLAY

Kids just want to have *fun*.

Youth sports surveys repeatedly show that youngsters would rather play a lot on a losing team than play very little on a winning team. Youth sports surveys repeatedly show that youngsters would rather play a lot on a losing team than play very little on a winning team. Youth sports surveys repeatedly show that youngsters would rather play a lot on a losing team than play very little on a winning team. Any questions? (That was a pure example of the principle of redundant repetition principle.) In other words, don't freak out if kids are less interested in winning; it is just their nature. In the earlier years, mental formation is developing over a sequence just like motor skills and body chemistry. Significant competition can throw a real wrench into that process if it becomes the main focus too early.

Application

Read closely, adults. Youngsters rarely view competition and games in the same cutthroat way that adults do. Adults play to win, even if it is a casual pickup game at lunch. They will risk a hamstring strain just to save the point. Killer instincts abound, testosterone is rampant, and we have all seen the adult who will beg, borrow, steal, or cheat to win. Children younger than 10 years view sports situations quite differently than adults. If left alone to play, kids take control of their own situations and do everything they can to keep a game close! They pick the teams and change them if they don't seem fair. If the rules make the game too complicated, they make new ones. If the score is becoming lopsided, they will alter the teams to even it up. Youngsters play for the sheer fun and experience of practicing new-found skills and being with their friends. Keeping in mind the child's point of view can help foster better experiences in activities without the need for strict, regimented rules.

One last time. Say it with me. Kids just want to have fun.

F. U. N.

Full **U**nlimited e**N**joyment.

★ ★ ★ ★ ★ ★ ★ ★ ★ ★ ★ ★ ★ ★ ★ ★ ★

SUCCESS RX

1. All 3 components of physical, chemical, and mental development are essential and cannot function maximally to your child's benefit without the other 2 in place.

2. Children's comparison activities to start forming ideas about themselves usually begin around age 5 years.

3. Being excited about an activity is a normal response; fear of an event is caused by significant stress. Having a strong definition of reality success can reduce fear of the outcome of an event.

4. Begin a habit of searching for positive and encouraging things to say to your child, and you can have an effect on self-esteem over time.

5. Viewpoints of youth sports participation center around increasing the emphasis on having fun and decreasing the emphasis on winning.

6. Youth sports surveys show that youngsters would rather play a lot on a losing team than play very little on a winning team. Children younger than 10 years view games and competition differently than adults.

7. Kids just want to have fun.

★ ★ ★ ★ ★ ★ ★ ★ ★ ★ ★ ★ ★ ★ ★ ★ ★

Between You and Me

1. Think about the patterns or rituals you are in the habit of doing and how you apply those to your child in sports and activities. Take the time to really look at the things your child does right in sports, school, and home, and mention those things first. Can you get in the new habit of encouraging your kids more often?

2. Remember that a little praise goes a long, long way in the eyes and ears of a child. You are helping your child form the basis of self-worth. That self-worth should not be a sport. That self-worth should be a human being living inside kid's clothes. What ways can you start or continue to positively impact your child's opinion of himself or herself long before entering into more competitive situations?

Mind Games

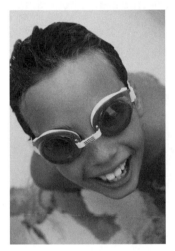

OK. Visualize this race. You can do this. Use good technique. Don't breathe too fast. Concentrate. Go hard at the end. Finish strong.

Sweaty palms. Stay calm. This is a fun race. I like this sport. Yeah, Joey is in this race, too, but I have worked really hard. But remember what happened last time—I got my best time and still only got second place.

"Go Johnny! Go fast!"

My parents are great. I really want to win, but if I don't, what will they do? I hope they won't be disappointed. They never seem to get upset, so I guess they won't start now. They are glad if I have tried to do everything right in my race, and don't really seem to care if I win. That's a big weight off my shoulders. Thank goodness, because I put enough weight on myself.

Young children progress through different developmental pathways that allow them to successfully maneuver through various skills, grasp basic and complex exercise techniques, improve their fitness, and participate in a variety of sports. The concepts in this book apply to your child who is involved in backyard play, PE class, recreational soccer, community league football, travel softball teams, varsity volleyball, or national-level golf. All of these experiences can be full of reality success and for that, I just encourage you to encourage your child to be *active.*

Sports are unfortunately synonymous with *intense competition* all too often. Kids can be involved in sports activities of all levels, have successful and gratifying experiences, yet not have the pressure of intense win-loss events. If they do choose to be active in more competitive sports and move on to an age and skill level at which competition is more appropriate, readiness to compete is influenced by mental and emotional development in addition to chemical maturation and motor improvement. If a good foundation of support has been laid, the house of self-esteem is sturdy and not easily huffed, puffed, and blown by windy big bad wolf pressures or shaken by stormy win-loss results. It is with this positive foundation that we see young athletes thrive on perfecting skill levels and competing because they really enjoy the recreational activities or sports in which they are participating.

Adolescents who are struggling for identity among their siblings or classmates may find a unique area of improvement and accomplishment in an activity such as a certain sport, musical instrument, or artistic performance, which causes their self-confidence to blossom.

If their identity becomes significantly associated with the sport or activity and they fail, however, their identity also can fail.

Parents who live through their child's accomplishments can fall into that dark pit and put excessive stress on the child to continue to perform without allowing any room for second place. Young athletes have young psychological makeup, so they cannot be treated like adult athletes. This is a point that cannot be emphasized enough. (Insert bells, whistles, and fireworks here.) Youth should not be placed in a significant or intense win-loss situation until they are confident that their worth is not based on the outcome of the athletic activity.

INSTANT REPLAY

Youth should not be placed in significant or intense win-loss situations until they are confident that their worth is not based on the outcome of the athletic activity.

The good news is that most children and adolescents play sports and compete without any long-term negative effects, and research shows that the large majority of children who are involved in sports do not suffer from excessive stress. However, there are important psychological bruises for the youngster who is placed in a sport that she is not interested in or ready for or is pushed too hard. Older athletes in later high school, college, national, Olympic, or professional sports strive to meet ambitiously high standards that they place on themselves. However, with few exceptions, young children and young athletes rarely display these traits unless there has been considerable influence and pressure from parents or coaches to accomplish certain goals.

INSTANT REPLAY

Young children rarely place overly high standards on themselves unless there has been considerable influence and pressure from parents or coaches to accomplish certain goals.

It is necessary and critical that youngsters participating in activities and sports be given opportunities to succeed as well as chances to have a successful outcome from an unsuccessful event. Reality sports success often comes from learning from previous failures! Reality success comes from youngsters bettering themselves no matter how they placed at the finish. Reality success comes from a positive sports or exercise experience in which they participate because it is pleasing, instead of participating to please everyone else. Thinking they can never fail does not give youngsters the chance to reach their full potential because they will always be intimidated or hold back just to be safe.

Part of the remedy for dealing with the ups and downs of the sports roller coaster involves knowing that every day will not be the same. Sometimes we can ride that roller coaster with our hands in the air; sometimes we can barely keep down our popcorn. So it is with sports and activities. Some days will feel good and much can be accomplished. Some days will just not click and performance will be lacking. But if each day is approached with the same attitude of always trying to improve technique and form and give the best effort no matter the result, each day of training or competition can be accepted as a successful event. Every day *is* different for everyone. That's reality. This approach can significantly affect an experience because the viewpoint is different than usual and avoids seeing down days as failures. Emphasis on the *effort* instead of winning must be modeled and taught by coaches and parents. This is rarely a concept youngsters figure out by themselves. Bravo to the ones who actually do!

INSTANT REPLAY

Emphasis on *effort* instead of winning must be modeled and taught to youngsters.

I have smiled as I see quotes on television, in magazines, and in newspapers from Olympic athletes who put these same points into reality. One points out that if he has done great by his own standards, he has done great. Even though his previous Olympic medals were silver, they were wins to him because his version of success is different from the standard version. Another emphasized that she wasn't going to try to be perfect anymore, just become better. Her goal is achieving her personal best because then she knows she has done everything possible, no matter the results. Even some world champions acknowledge that society has become obsessed with the gold medal instead of great personal achievements.

Another way to enhance involvement in an activity is to let your kid experience different activities and eventually gravitate toward the ones she most enjoys. How many of us like breakfast buffets? I see those hands. The wide world of sports from the pinnacle of success to the agony of defeat should be seen as a big smorgasbord for kids to try various kinds and even go back for seconds. There are many youth who attach themselves to a sport early on and specialize without trying many other sports. This early specialization can be a positive experience without problems if there has not been parental pressure or unrealistic expectations to be confined to one sport. Your Jackie may be a star at 13 years of age and love her sport. That is wonderful, as long as she is not pressured and has an identity outside of the sport. Obviously, I see many talented youth who start narrowing their sports focus before puberty and have a wonderful outcome. For every one of those who are ahead of the developmental schedule, however, there are significantly more children who will benefit from delaying true specialization.

As I have mentioned previously, young bodies subjected to extreme training regimens or excessive training hours are perfect targets for overuse injuries. Tremendous time away from family and friends during competition or many hours of training requires extra effort on your part as parents to spend quality time with Johnny rather than as Johnny the athlete. It is crucial that your child have help establishing his or her identity separate from the sport. Reports from some athletes who became world champions at early ages reveal a huge psychological adjustment when their worlds and self-images no longer revolved around their sport.

Burnout is an increasingly concerning consequence of the stress and pressure put on our youth today. There is a serious difference between burnout and stopping a sport for other reasons. Kids may want to stop a sport, and that is not necessarily a bad thing. If they have given a reasonable effort and time commitment and still do not want to continue, it is probably time to try another sport. Think about how long we adults stick with something we are not interested in the next time you pick up the television remote—a few seconds, maybe?

Youngsters will often stop or quit a sport if they are not having an enjoyable experience, they do not feel a sense of accomplishment, their reason for participating changes (such as friends stopping the sport), or simply another activity attracts their attention. Quitting an activity to transfer to another sport is very common and can be a healthy decision. This transfer has the value of exposure to other sports and allows youngsters to see which activities are enjoyable and give them a sense of accomplishment. One of our world's best female figure skaters started in gymnastics and then switched to skating at 7 years of age after trying it with one of her friends. Not a bad decision, huh?

INSTANT REPLAY

Children will stop or quit a sport or activity if they are not enjoying it, do not feel a sense of accomplishment, change their reason for participating, or become attracted to another activity.

Most youth involved in sports and recreational activities reap many benefits and do not experience excessive stress. Sad situations include youth who are pressured to do a sport, stay in a sport to gain the attention of their parents, have unrealistic expectations to live up to, get frequent overuse injuries, or are loved conditionally by their win-loss record. If they do not feel they are able to satisfy these impossible demands, the activity no longer becomes enjoyable and athletes start to experience burnout and lose interest. Other risk factors associated with burnout include youth who are exceptionally perfectionistic, have high self-imposed expectations, have lower self-esteem, maintain a "win at all costs" attitude, train long hours with little variation, or experience inconsistent coaching. If parents and coaches understand and recognize these risk factors, hopefully a bad outcome can be avoided.

If self-esteem and communication skills are not optimal, youth who are not enjoying an activity may find it extremely difficult to communicate that feeling to their parents or coaches, so make every effort to communicate effectively with your child. Altered or unhealthy behavior in the child should be a warning sign. If young athletes start showing evidence that they are not interested in going to practice or excited about an upcoming competition or if they start acting out of character, pay attention.

Doctors, coaches, and parents need to be aware of potential red flags when a sports-injured youth does not get better with appropriate therapy at the expected rate, has a poor response to treatment that is out of proportion to the original injury, or repeatedly has a setback just before or after being cleared to return to participation.

Identifying these situations is important because physical or medical treatment of the injury is not solving the source of the problem. There may be secondary motivation behind the behavior, such as

- Inability to communicate a desire to change sports
- Saving face for a poor performance
- Avoidance of competition because of fear of failure
- Wanting to remain dependent on parents
- Securing the attention of parents

Adolescents and children may be overwhelmed by the demands of training and performance, so an injury can offer a socially accepted way of escape. Unfortunately, using this type of avoidance does not allow for full functioning or performing to the child's potential.

INSTANT REPLAY

Adolescents and children may be overwhelmed by the demands of training and performance, so an injury can offer a socially accepted way of escape—but this type of avoidance does not allow for full functioning or reaching full potential.

Many parents are fantastic private detectives about their children's lives—how do parents always have eyes in the back of their heads?—but are farsighted when it comes to their children having problems in their activities or sports. Pay careful attention to detect changes in desire or activity patterns. Parents should not be distracted by their own desires for the child to participate. Take off the blinders. Step back. Look at the whole situation. Set aside your desires for a moment.

Talk to your young, active child. Unconditional support and established value in your child independent of competitive sports can save a young mind and body from a lot of pressure. Coaches are often witness to problems because they are on the front lines and may see the changes first. In either case, please do not wait for the situation to become out of hand before addressing a potential problem.

INSTANT REPLAY

Unconditional support and established value in your child independent of competitive sports can save a young mind and body from a lot of pressure.

Application

A strong sense of self. A strong sense of competence. A strong sense of accomplishment. These ideals keep children and youth interested in continuing to participate. It should be our goal as adults to find ways to make that continuation happen. Support and encouragement from parents and coaches can aid in producing positive experiences in sports activities. If that is the case, there are fewer boundaries for enjoyment and a healthy view of fitness, sports, and exercise. Performance potential can be maximized and multiple lifelong benefits can occur—enhanced levels of fitness, increased self-esteem and confidence, heightened qualities of discipline and leadership, and improved overall performance in school, family, work, and life.

★ ★ ★ ★ ★ ★ ★ ★ ★ ★ ★ ★ ★ ★ ★ ★ ★

SUCCESS RX

1. If a good foundation of support has been laid, children can thrive on improving skills and competing because they really enjoy the activities in which they are participating.

2. Youth should not be placed in significant or intense win-loss situations until they are confident that their worth is not based on the outcome of the activity.

3. It is necessary that youngsters participating in activities be given opportunities to have reality success by experiencing accomplishment as well as learning from mistakes.

4. If each day is approached with the same attitude of improving technique and giving one's best effort no matter the result, each day of participation can be accepted as a successful event because every day is different for everyone.

5. Stopping an activity to transfer to another one grants more exposure to different sports and allows kids to see which activities are enjoyable and give them a sense of accomplishment.

6. Make every effort to have good communication with your children to know what they like and don't like about their sports and activities.

7. A strong sense of self, competence, and accomplishment keeps youth interested in continuing to participate in exercise and sports.

★ ★ ★ ★ ★ ★ ★ ★ ★ ★ ★ ★ ★ ★ ★ ★ ★

Between You and Me

1. It is always amazing that children can have such different personalities even when they are in the same family. Do you have a particular child with personality traits that may make him or her at higher risk for more stress with competition? If so, how can you start to accommodate that with a supportive environment?

2. Remember that a desire to change or stop an activity is not necessarily a bad thing. Listen to your child's thoughts about that activity to see if it becomes more evident what the change is all about. Are you willing to let your child change, or do you want him or her to stay in it because it is the sport you want?

3. Sitting down and having an adult conversation with your child may be difficult. Kids may talk better when you are doing something fun with them that they enjoy. What are some creative ways you can improve the level of communication between you and your child?

Accessories for Success

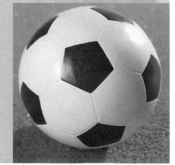

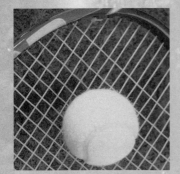

Fat, Phat, or Fanatic

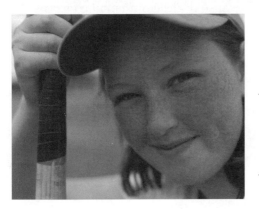

Now that I am involved in more activities, I get to see just how different we all are! I couldn't possibly try to be like everybody else, so I will just continue to do my best. I feel for some of my friends, though. Justin is struggling a lot because he is so big and heavy. He finally decided to do sports and not care what anyone else thinks, but he has to work so hard.

Then there's Janice, who works so hard and never stops. I get tired just watching her. It's hard for her to be consistent because it seems like she is always coming back from an injury. Why does she get hurt so much?

Welcome to the section on accessories for success. I want to include some important things that can have a profound effect on whether a youngster can have a successful and positive experience with activities. The

4 areas that will be in this section are overweight and obesity, over-training and overuse injuries, nutrition, and strength training.

Exercise for overweight kids is an excellent intervention, but it must be approached carefully because of developmental concerns and risk of overuse injury.

INSTANT REPLAY

> Exercise for overweight youth is an excellent intervention, but it must be approached carefully because of developmental concerns and risk of overuse injury.

The obesity epidemic is somewhat paralleled by the rising appearance of overuse injuries in children and teens. These injuries invade the exercise or sports experience and often occur because children are being pushed beyond their developmental capabilities. Nutrition plays a role in providing necessary support for exercise and growth in this unique time of life when the body changes so quickly, and strength training has the potential to add participation value if used within appropriate limitations.

In this chapter, I hope to provide you with some insight to the sensitive issue of kids who are overweight and the out-of-control issue of kids who are overtrained. Certainly there are health and sports implications for these situations and yes, development is also involved. I know there are people out there who have good intentions to help kids lose weight and become more physically fit, but if kids who are overweight are approached the same way as kids who are not, many of those overweight youth end up in my clinic with an overuse injury. Don't get me wrong—exercise, proper nutrition, and surrounding environment are all important for addressing this issue. What I want to do is examine the exercise component from a sports medicine point of view and show why it is not as easy as it seems. If you have a child who is overweight or even obese, I hope this information will give you more assistance in providing fun, safe, and injury-free guidance for a transition into exercise that is filled with reality success.

Balance is the key, just like it is with many things in life. Sure, kids should have some time to relax and not be on the run every hour of every day, but they do need time to be physically active. Balancing activities plays a significant role in keeping a child from experiencing too much pressure while trying to enjoy some sort of exercise or sport. Exercise should not be forced or used as punishment or disciplinary action, but should be spoken of positively and encouraged. Parents who participate in regular exercise of some kind offer good role models of a lifelong approach to and positive outlook on exercise. Doing family activities together not only gives everyone an exercise opportunity, but also builds family bonds and helps enrich the attitude toward exercise, fitness, and long-term health.

OK, so what is the big deal about exercising or not exercising, being active or inactive? Big deal? Let me tell you about big deal. We have multiple extras that come from living in a land of opportunity. One of those is extra food. Another is being able to enjoy many things from the couch. Extra food plus extra time not being active equals extra weight. This information isn't just media hype. The

President's Council on Physical Fitness and Sports has seen a trend over time that shows our youth having lower levels of fitness and higher levels of body fat than youth of many years ago. Millions of our youth younger than 19 years are overweight. Many already have risk factors for heart disease and other health problems like diabetes associated with overweight and obesity. With all the available opportunities for activities ranging from recreational to team sports, one would think that rising obesity isn't logical. But it does make sense when you look at it closely. Kids have just as much opportunity to be sedentary as they do to be active. We must not forget that some youngsters do not have genetics on their side and battle with weight problems despite diet and exercise. At the same time, the majority of youth who have been bitten by the bulge are usually members of the 3-T club—television, technology, and taste buds.

INSTANT REPLAY

Kids have just as much opportunity to be sedentary as they do to be active.

It has been shown in many research publications that the risk of obesity increases greatly with each hour of television watched. Reducing the amount of time watching television and removing the television from a child's room can have a positive effect on fighting inactivity. The same goes for technology. I can't imagine surviving without e-mail, a computer, and the Internet, so I truly appreciate the value of technology. At the same time, hours spent playing video or computer games can have a similar effect on your child's weight. Our society caters to our taste buds, and sometimes I think the new basic 4 food groups have become buffet, dine in, carryout, and delivery—not to mention that a huge pile of food on a plate is some kids' idea of the revised Food Pyramid. Excess sugary foods, poor portion control, and unhealthy fat contents all contribute to our problematic size scenario.

Overweight and Obesity

People are finally starting to see the light and realize the serious effects of being overweight on our young population. This awareness will hopefully make a difference in their future. Children are getting risk factors for heart disease, fatty deposits in their blood vessels, high levels of cholesterol, and dramatic increases in type 2 diabetes— which used to be called adult-onset diabetes because it was not seen in kids. Well, no longer are those health problems reserved for adults. Another issue is the effect on self-esteem and the psychological well-being of the child. And the longer a child stays overweight, the greater the chance he will remain that way as an adult. Once he becomes an overweight parent, he often starts a similar cycle with his own children. It is important for us all to try to help break that unhealthy cycle.

INSTANT REPLAY

The longer a child stays overweight, the greater the chance he or she will remain that way as an adult.

The American Academy of Pediatrics, a major child advocate organization made up of more than 60,000 pediatricians across the country, has made reducing the problem of overweight children one of its top priorities. Unfortunately, just as the number of overweight youngsters is rising, the opportunities for PE classes in public schools are declining. Many schools have dropped PE classes because of financial problems, while others just do not have the staff available. Some schools have quit requiring PE for graduation. Even the schools that do have such classes may not be optimal situations because many of the kids spend a large part of class time getting changed, waiting in line for their turn, and getting dressed again. We must all do our part to stop the insanity and help our children as well as ourselves get some form of exercise. Thankfully, there is growing research and a rising number of programs available to help form some guidance to solving the nationwide weight problem. Some school programs and PE teachers are making great headway by focusing their classes more on fitness-related activities than just playing games and are finding ways to creatively increase the time your kids are actually active.

This crossroad is where some of the problem lies. For some reason, society often emphasizes the importance of competition and winning rather than exercise itself. This does not help a youngster feel good about getting even a low to moderate amount of exercise and may often lead to guilt about not wanting to compete on a structured team sport. We have got to change that attitude and encourage activity at any level as a positive healthy behavior. Walking the dog briskly, riding the bike to the store, playing tag in the backyard, and participating on a team are all acceptable forms of exercise. Getting 45 to 60 minutes of activity on as many days as possible, even if it is broken up into 15-minute segments, is an important and achievable goal. Not all kids have to be in organized sports, but the health statistics show that kids need to be doing something or we will all be in trouble with medical bills.

Overuse and Overtraining

Now the yin and the yang—just when you thought it was safe to exercise…. The childhood overweight epidemic is a major problem in the United States without question. However, there is another major iceberg that has appeared on the opposite end of the horizon, and that is too much exercise. Yes, it's those terrible toos again—too much obesity and too many injuries from too much pressure to exercise too much. Two major crises in our young population—obesity *and* overuse injuries. Who knew? Such a dilemma. We have kids pounding their faces with chips and kids pounding their bodies on the pavement. Two situations that need to find a happy medium. In our zeal to promote exercise, it is crucial to avoid falling into the societal trap of pushing kids too much once they are involved in sports or exercise activities.

On one spectrum, there are too many youngsters with a weight problem who need exercise. On the other hand, there are too many youngsters with an overexercise problem who need to cut back. It's the "battle of the bulge with those who overindulge," if you will. There is a substantial rise in the number of overuse injuries in our younger, active population. Just like we have kids with health problems once confined to adults, we also have injuries previously confined to adults that are now trickling down into our active youth. As kids start increasing the intensity and duration of training to adult levels, adult-type injuries begin to appear. I have noticed a substantial increase in the number and severity of youth sports injuries in my practice over the past few years. Some of these injuries are fractures, ligament tears, and concussions that are often hard to avoid, but many of the injuries are caused by outright overuse and inappropriate training. High levels of intense exercise and repetition in a young, growing body can lead to some undesirable results, especially if the increased training stems from excessive pressure or a lack of knowledge about skill development and maturation.

INSTANT REPLAY

There is a substantial rise in the number of overuse injuries in our younger, active population.

In my profession of pediatric and adolescent sports medicine, it is heartbreaking for me to see a 13-year-old gymnast almost at Olympic level have to end her career because of multiple overuse injuries, or an elite 12-year-old figure skater who stops her career short with a stress fracture in her leg after being spoken of as "one of the best to come along in years." The list goes on and is always sad to see. Kids this young with ability and talent should not have to produce world-class performances at that age. Congratulations if they can, but what is the insatiable drive behind us having to see mere children achieve athletic feats at younger and younger ages? Sometimes nobody is to blame. Overuse injuries are not always from a pushy parent or coach making the athlete train excessively. Some of these injuries are caused merely by the fact that the child is in love with the sport, everyone sees potential, and the young athlete is allowed to train far more than a young body is capable of sustaining.

Of the millions of youth in our country, there is a very positive increase in the number of kids involved in exercise or sports activity. Remember, though, that there are huge numbers of estimated injuries, many of which are caused by overuse, that should be *preventable.* Even though it is hard to know the exact numbers, I would bet that with the amount of overuse injuries that do show up in my clinic, the true numbers must be staggering.

Sure, your child gets hurt in the backyard, at recess, and in sports. Somehow, though, injuries from sports have become more socially acceptable compared with other forms of injuries. There is no doubt that injuries do occur in activities and sports and are often just bad luck. Overuse injuries, on the flip side, should be under more control because they often occur after a significant increase in activity. If such large numbers of injuries are potentially preventable because they are caused by too much intense exercise by young bodies, this area should not be overlooked. Families may view that type of injury proudly as a sign of their child's athletic ability, but those injuries will not look so good when they turn into arthritis at 45 or are covered up by a scar from knee replacement surgery later on—and then who is the one living with that consequence?

INSTANT REPLAY

> Overuse injuries are potentially preventable because they are caused by too much intense activity or too rapid an increase in activity.

So, too little exercise, too much exercise…is there a happy medium? Exercise must be encouraged, but in our society, sports have become synonymous with competition, winning, and fame. (Where do you see fitness, health, and fun in that list?) Everybody wants their children to be the star athletes, the youngest star athletes, the most successful athletes, the athletes with the best scholarships to the best universities with the best sports teams, and hopefully the athletes to obtain that coveted world medal or professional sports paycheck. Somehow they must think that their children's success will make other people see them as better parents. Think about it. Cavemen beat their chests; we shouldn't.

With the extreme amount of focus placed on being first—and anything less being failure—it is no wonder that pressure to perform starts at earlier ages. It becomes ingrained. It becomes the norm. It becomes accepted. Our competitive nature drives us to want to be the best. That desire by itself is healthy and allows most of us to accomplish many of our life goals and have a wonderful sense of self-worth. Yet it is easy to see how that principle can become distorted very quickly, especially if the adult mentors to our youth are doing the distorting.

OK. Can we talk? As a youth sports medicine specialist, I still say that part of the reason for this overuse and over-push phenomenon is simply a lack of knowledge. I think many people have great intentions, but just do not know what a body goes through to blossom athletically at any level. Kids are not adults in kids' clothing, so learning about how they are different can have a huge effect on their achievement and health and provide them with a positive sports experience and reality success. Much effort is needed from everyone to understand what pressures and influences are on your kids, why kids can or cannot do certain things at certain ages, and that too much exercise stress on a young, growing body can cause injury. Hopefully this understanding will decrease unnecessary stress on children and adults, encourage youth that exercise is good at all levels, prevent unrealistic expectations from parents and coaches, keep parents from achieving vicariously through their children, and decrease the number of overuse injuries in our young athletes. Knowledge is like gold. Not everyone has a lot, but what they have is very valuable.

INSTANT REPLAY

Much effort is needed from everyone to understand what pressures and influences are on your kids, why kids can or cannot do certain things at certain ages, and that too much exercise stress on a young, growing body can cause injury.

Overweight and Overuse

Let's bring these 2 together now and see how overweight and overuse are linked. Obesity has reached epidemic proportions, but people often do not realize that pushing your kids to overuse injuries has also reached similar epidemic proportions. Many overweight children are randomly thrown onto sports teams or into exercise programs and the same thing happens—they get pushed too quickly and end up with an overuse injury. These poor youngsters have now become part of not only 1, but 2 epidemic groups. It takes special guidance to respond to the challenge to help overweight kids slowly begin the process of adapting to exercise. With the 2 extremes on the exercise continuum, we seem to find ourselves somewhere between fat, phat, and fanatic. Balance becomes important to take advantage of the advancing progress of skill development without overloading the process during its course.

INSTANT REPLAY

Many overweight children are thrown onto sports teams or into exercise activity too quickly and end up with an overuse injury.

It takes special guidance to respond to the challenge to help overweight kids slowly begin the process of adapting to exercise.

In a perfect world, obesity and overuse injuries would not exist, but because that is not the world of kids I see, awareness and knowledge of how to avoid these problems becomes your vaccination against them. In previous years, sports and obesity were words rarely seen in the same sentence. Now with the national push to combat the overweight problem, more people are turning to exercise activities and sports for help. It is very important to understand that overweight children do pose specific challenges physically and developmentally. If they start a new activity to become more active and are treated just like every other youngster in that activity, the result may be an overuse injury and a defeated attempt to learn healthy lifestyle patterns. The focus of exercise and fitness in overweight youth differs from adults and from other non-overweight youth, and exercise programs should reflect that difference to help prevent a negative outcome and produce a positive experience.

Application

Let's bring you to some familiar territory—development. As you have seen, skills for youth sports activities mature over a sequential contin-uum. Part of the challenge with overweight or obese youngsters is they may have had very little previous exposure to sports or exercise and may lack sufficient skill development for their age. I don't think this situation is appreciated enough because it puts overweight youth at risk for an injury if placed in a situation in which it is just assumed the child is old enough to possess the skills necessary to participate in that activity. They can also be at risk for overuse injuries if they are pushed too hard to catch up to a certain skill level. Think about this in light of our discussions on skill maturation. You can't just flip a switch.

Remember that late bloomers who reach puberty later than their friends can be at a higher injury risk because of immature bones as well as deficits in strength and size. If your teenager is a late bloomer and also overweight, he may look like he has the ability to protect himself. Unfortunately, a lack of skills plus skeletal immaturity will still increase the risk of injury and reduce the chance for a positive experience when participating with peers that are more advanced physically and technically. Overweight youth who have the desire to participate, become more active, and increase their fitness should also be given the opportunity for more instruction on skills and the appropriate time to improve and build on those skills. Then you have the pieces in place to create a situation of reality success, encouragement, accomplishment, and a desire to continue.

Extra precautions should be taken when preparing an overweight youngster for an exercise or sports program. Significant weight can predispose a child to certain injuries or mechanical problems. A condition called slipped capital femoral epiphysis is the most common hip disorder in overweight and obese kids 10 to 18 years of age. I don't expect you to be able to pronounce it 3 times fast, but what happens is the growth plate of the hip literally slides off the bone like ice cream off of a cone, causing the child to limp, lose hip range of motion, and have referred pain to the thigh and knee. It is an important problem to be aware of because surgical correction is necessary. Overweight kids are often knock-kneed and have feet arches that flatten. They are often less flexible because of a lack of activity and often have poor strength for their size. These factors can all contribute to problems such as knee pain or shin splints if activities are advanced too quickly or involve a lot of impact. So simply telling an overweight child to "just go jog" may not be the best first step, so to speak. Poor mechanics and skill development, plus excess weight, plus rapid increase in activity, equals tissue overload. This type of situation is what we should all avoid, so youth can have a positive experience that continues to progress rather than one that discourages them from continuing.

Placing an overweight youngster in an exercise situation also poses a challenge in terms of the environment. I have already discussed the major chemical developments that occur in kids and make them very different from adults, such as poor sweating mechanisms, thirst drives, and adaptation to the heat. Being overweight or obese adds more risk to the situation. Larger body mass requires more energy to move, thus generating more heat, especially coupled with inefficient movements because of a lack of skill development. Higher fat content retains more heat, making it more risky for a youngster that already has poor heat-lowering ability.

Because beginning fitness level is often low in a child who is overweight, a substantial amount of time may be necessary to progress basic fitness levels to more advanced levels of exercise. Extra time is also important to acquire skills and technique necessary for safe activity. Decreasing inactivity-induced inflexibility with stretching and adding strength to inactive muscles can improve an overall exercise situation. Strength training may help to burn some calories and increase metabolic rate when combined with nonimpact or low-impact aerobic activities. The onset of exercise must be gradual to allow time to improve skill acquisition as well as adapt to the new energy requirements and demands on their body tissues.

Following heart rate is good to show youngsters that they are actually exercising, and they should be rewarded based on self-improvement and accomplishment, rather than how quickly they finish compared to other kids. It is also important to not obsess about watching the scales. As body composition changes occur, the changes on the scale may not be as impressive. It may be more helpful to follow successful changes in body composition or body mass index specific for age and gender, if available. Thinking of ways to monitor effort and reward that effort takes creativity, but is worth it to encourage these kids. Exercise programs for overweight youngsters must be individualized because the same developmental pathways apply, but may be delayed or take longer to learn. If the whole family can be involved, it can help the child feel less isolated and also provide reality success for more people. If you are a parent or coach of an overweight child, please take into consideration these principles to provide reduced risk for overuse injuries and a positive activity experience.

The goal of activity is to help an overweight child or teen be encouraged to continue exercising in a fitness program or sport without being pushed too hard, too quickly. Overweight or obese children and teens who are thrown into exercise programs or sports often rapidly end up with injuries that defeat the purpose. We must be very careful not to take them from one epidemic group and place them into another. All kids deserve a positive activity experience that will encourage them to sustain a lifetime of healthy habits, good nutrition, and fitness. There are 2 extremes—obesity and overuse—and we need to find the right middle ground because it is much better to be phat than fat or a fanatic.

★ ★ ★ ★ ★ ★ ★ ★ ★ ★ ★ ★ ★ ★ ★

SUCCESS RX

1. The epidemic of overweight and obesity is somewhat paralleled by the rising appearance of overuse injuries in children and teens.

2. Parents who participate in regular exercise of some kind offer good role models of a lifelong approach and positive outlook on exercise.

3. The risk of overweight and obesity increases greatly with each hour of television watched. We must encourage activity at any level as a positive healthy behavior. Getting 45 to 60 minutes of activity on as many days as possible, even if broken up into segments, is an important and achievable goal.

4. Just like we have kids with health problems once confined to adults, we also have injuries previously confined to adults that are now trickling down into our active youth as more of them are trained with adult levels of intensity and duration.

5. Understanding development can decrease unnecessary stress on children and adults, encourage youth that exercise is good at all levels, prevent unrealistic expectations from parents and coaches, keep parents from achieving vicariously through their children, and decrease the number of overuse injuries in our youngsters.

6. The focus of exercise and fitness in overweight youth differs from adults and from other non-overweight youth, and exercise programs should reflect that difference to help prevent a negative outcome and produce a positive experience.

7. Overweight youth may lack sufficient skill development for their age and need more instruction and time to improve those skills. They can be at risk for overuse injuries if pushed too hard to catch up to a certain skill level.

8. Significant weight can predispose a child to certain injuries or mechanical problems and adds more risk for problems with adapting to the heat. The onset of exercise must be gradual to allow time to improve skill acquisition as well as adapt to new energy requirements and demands on their body.

★ ★ ★ ★ ★ ★ ★ ★ ★ ★ ★ ★ ★ ★ ★ ★

Between You and Me

1. The number of children and teenagers who are significantly overweight is staggering. Having exposure to exercise and activity opportunities are important to help promote a healthy lifestyle. What are you doing to positively promote exercise and activity in your family?

2. Maybe you have a child who is overweight. Maybe you have one who exercises too much. Neither situation is optimal. Where does your child fall on the exercise scale, and how can you help steer her or him to a better middle ground?

3. Improving fitness and health in an overweight youngster can be challenging. It is important to understand the factors involved that can allow activity without increasing the risk of an overuse injury or a negative outcome. How can you take a family approach to proper exercise, good nutrition, and weight control?

Breakfast, Lunch, and Dinner of Champions

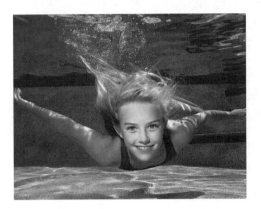

I am always hungry! Mom and Dad laugh because I eat double what my younger brother and sister eat. They tell me it's because I have to fill in those extra 5 inches I grew last year. Sometimes I feel too full when I am going to play my sports; other days I can hardly run because I don't have any energy. I don't understand what I should be eating or taking. I see Joey take a handful of pills and Jimmy drinking some special drink. I don't really see any difference when they play. I went to the store the other day with my Mom, and there were so many bottles on the shelves that I got dizzy just looking at all of them!

Working with young athletes from beginners to Olympians, I have had the opportunity to see the positive benefits of exercise and competition, and also the poor outcomes from excessive pressures to perform. In this day and age, there are more opportunities for kids to be active and in sports, which is a good thing, but as with most good things, they can get distorted with increased pressures to perform. Some of this distortion shows up in the way athletes try to fuel themselves nutritionally by eating or swallowing anything they think will give them an edge. I am amazed many times with what they put into their mouths without really knowing much about the substance. They just heard about it from a friend, read about it in a fitness magazine, or saw a competitor taking it. So I guess that makes it work? Sounds pretty shaky to me—and pretty dangerous. Nutritional fads and supplement use are rampant among our youth, yet there is often very little information to back up a lot of the claims of the supplement companies. With all the new expensive equipment, positive drug tests, and personal trainers, it is clear that parents, coaches, and athletes are all looking for some kind of an advantage.

INSTANT REPLAY

Nutritional fads and supplement use are rampant among our youth, yet often there is very little information to really back up a lot of the claims from the supplement companies.

Supplements

Often athletic kids and their parents and coaches feel that adequate training, good technique, good recovery, and sound nutrition are just not enough for the ultimate performance they want. These recommendations just don't sound sexy enough, while the latest supplement does. Not too long ago, supplement use in young athletes was primarily limited to protein pills and shakes taken by high school football players to gain weight. Unfortunately, now we are faced with the challenges and dangers of the use of anabolic steroids, even in middle school. The use of other supplements has skyrocketed as young athletes succumb to the pressures of winning at any cost, even their lives. Many youth will watch what wealthy sports stars endorse. Unfortunately, money does not provide immortality, and kids as well as adults are putting their health at risk. It is frequent practice for athletes to operate under the motto that if a little is good, more can be better. There is little research to show what happens when these products are used by adults, and no research to show what happens at young ages in rapidly growing bodies. Many supplements on the market just don't have the research to give their proposed results scientific credibility, yet people are swayed by the "next best thing" phenomenon. A doctor friend of mine told me that supplements are causing a new syndrome. You may have heard of it. I'm sure you've seen it. He calls it the supplement stare. You walk into a store and suddenly it's very, very quiet. Everyone is frozen—gazing at thousands of little bottles that start to blur into one. Be careful—it might be contagious.

Before supplements, athletes relied on food. Then supplements showed up along with illegal performance-enhancing drugs. Those are obviously still a big problem. There is an amazing amount of money—billion$ of dollar$—spent on supplements to gain muscle, lose body fat, and improve performance. The majority of dietary supplements are not reviewed by the Food and Drug Administration and they arrive on the market so quickly that true medical research lags way behind in its attempts to weed out the ones that work from the ones that don't. Needless to say, you should always do your homework and be very hesitant for your youngster to take supplements when potential or actual side effects are unknown for actively growing bodies. It would take another entire book to go through all of the supplements out there, so instead I will try to bring us back to the basics of what exercise entails, what the body needs, and how good nutrition can help enhance exercise and sports performance.

What about vitamins? For years, I had the bottle on my kitchen table without even questioning if they were helpful. I have come to realize that certain vitamins are critical for body functions, immune system effectiveness, and antioxidant protection, but the *source* of those vitamins is the crucial point. There is a concept called *bioavailability,* which refers to how effectively something is used by the body. Try to find independent bioavailability research on a particular supplement or vitamin and you may be looking for a long, long time. Synthetic vitamins are isolated or fragmented nutrients and the body is not as effective at using them in that form, even if they are cleverly disguised as a cereal flake. I tend to think that is why more and more vitamin bottles boast about packing in a lot more than the daily required amount. That may help explain why you or your child might have the most expensive and yellow urine in town. Even more concerning is the fact that there have been large research studies that have investigated the effects of certain vitamins and found that in some cases, those synthetic vitamins caused more harm than good. *Food,* on the other hand, contains great sources of those same vitamins in natural forms that are not isolated or fragmented. Fresh raw fruits and vegetables contain vitamins that are combined with more than 10,000 plant chemicals and enzymes, all of which work together to help the body effectively and efficiently use them. So if you want some vitamin C, I would look a lot more closely at that orange in the fruit bowl on your table rather than just seeing it as decoration. Foods may contain less actual vitamin content than a pill, but they are much more available and effective for the body to use—a basic concept of quality versus quantity.

What about protein? There are times when a little extra protein is actually appropriate. During the rapid growth phase of puberty, extra protein is needed to help sustain growth of body tissues. In sports that are strength or endurance based, it appears that the daily requirement is slightly increased, but only by a small amount, so handfuls of horse-sized protein pills may be over the top.

Overcoming Tissue Damage and Stress Chemicals Associated With Exercise

If we are going to discuss the role of nutrition in exercise, it is important to first discuss the different aspects of exercise that can benefit from good nutrition—overcoming tissue damage and stress chemicals and providing fuel for exercise at all levels. Our bodies are incredibly capable of handling and adapting to exercise. Microscopic breakdown occurs every day, which your body repairs during rest with the use of healthy tissues and good nutrients. However, if the breakdown is not able to completely repair before the next bout of exercise demand, it starts to exceed the repair, and an overuse injury begins to form. This is the common scenario in which exercise or training is too intense or too often without proper recovery time. You know, the paper clip theory—keep bending it and it will break.

During intense exercise activity and any associated emotional stress, a process occurs called *oxidative stress,* during which the body produces chemical by-products such as cortisol and free radicals. Consider these by-products the exhaust produced by your car engine. These chemicals are *catabolic,* which means they are more likely to break down or damage tissues in the body instead of build them up. This isn't an organic chemistry class, but let's just say that all of the processes happening in the body to produce the energy output required for exercise also produce bad waste products that need to be cleared from the body. We don't have chimneys to clear that smoke, so our bodies must rely on other means to clear them.

INSTANT REPLAY

During intense exercise activity and any associated emotional stress, a process occurs called *oxidative stress,* during which the body produces chemical by-products such as free radicals.

If the production of these chemicals is too high and exercise is too intense, this combination can have a negative effect on the good tissues of the body, causing damage to our DNA, muscle soreness, poor recovery from exercise, and a progressive decline in performance. Inability of the body to recover also overstresses the immune system, allowing infections to strike when the body is vulnerable. Excess free radicals are basically scavengers that steal valuable ingredients necessary for body repair, recovery, and energy production. Ways to help reduce this oxidative stress and free radical production include

- Spread out highly intense exercise bouts.
- Allow sufficient recovery time.
- Get adequate rest.
- Stay well hydrated.
- Have daily nutrition that is high in antioxidants, which directly fight free radicals (the body's Pac-Man effect).

Antioxidants are found in foods with high sources of vitamin C, vitamin E, beta-carotene, and phytochemicals (plant chemicals) such as raw, colorful fruits and vegetables. These nutritional sources are absolutely necessary for the athletic or active individual.

Providing Fuel for Exercise

Because many common supplements cannot be supported, recommended, or proven to be completely safe in youth—and often are ineffective, temporary, or dangerous—it is important to rely on the gold standards of training, technique, and nutrition. Good, solid nutritional practices have been promoted by some as the best sports supplement in existence. Unlike supplements, food is effective, perpetual, and safe.

INSTANT REPLAY

Good nutrition has been promoted by some as the best sports supplement in existence.

There is no doubt that appropriate nutritional status is a prime factor in allowing a body to perform at its best potential. I have seen world-class athletes with all the talent in the world consistently perform poorly with a horrifying nutritional regimen until they finally realize that good nutrition is fundamentally as important to their training as lifting weights and practicing. I think they often see their achievements as unaffected by their nutrition and that if they are a world-record holder living off of fries, chips, burgers, soft drinks, and ice cream, they are still a world-record holder. But how much better could they possibly perform if their cells were all more nutritionally healthy? I can't give that answer, but logic says that their performance could reach a higher potential if their entire body was firing on all cylinders.

Finding the right balance of proteins, carbohydrates, and healthy fats seems to be the rage today, but there is no denying that youngsters in general and those in exercise activities need well-balanced nutrition that includes them all. In addition to the right balance, it's also important to make healthy food choices, such as complex carbohydrates and grains, as well as "good" fats and omega-3 fatty acids. Even fluids are extremely important and often overlooked as a valuable resource for training and competition. For instance, it has been shown that with as little as 2% to 3% dehydration, performance is significantly affected in a negative way.

INSTANT REPLAY

Performance can be significantly affected by as little as 2% to 3% dehydration.

Proper nutrition is critically important to sustain activity, exercise, and training requirements. In kids, tremendous calories are required to grow and build important body tissues as well as fuel exercise demands. That's why multiple smaller meals and healthy snacks are better than spacing out the basic 3 meals a day. Their bodies need refueling much more often than that. Nutrition provides the body with the ability to not only sustain exercise and training, but also provide fuel for recovery and refueling after energy has been used. This chapter is not intended to give out detailed and specific nutritional meal plans, but rather to give a broad view of general nutritional concepts and explain how development even plays a role.

General Concepts of Nutrition

Good nutrition—it's not just for breakfast anymore. It's for growth of a young body, preventing diseases, maintaining healthy functioning tissues of the body all the way to your cells, and fueling the body involved in exercise activity. Daily proper nutrition helps sustain and support exercise demands on a regular basis. If your child participates in competitions or sporting events, there are some more basics to cover.

Pre-event nutrition. Remember that the days leading up to an event or practice are important to keep fuel and energy stores full with good sources of complex carbohydrates. Fats are slow and difficult to digest, so they should be avoided for the few hours before an event. Choose good sources of nutrition that the body can use quickly without the danger of a sugar crash. A donut with a candy bar chaser is not the way to go—but don't think I haven't seen it.

Maintaining excellent hydration is also key to prevent going into an event already dry.

During-event nutrition. Fluids such as water and sports drinks are important to maintain energy and hydration. If the event lasts for hours with breaks between competition, light carbohydrate snacks such as fruit, natural yogurts, or concentrated gels can be used along with water and sports drinks. Highly caffeinated drinks or high-sugar soft drinks are not recommended because these pull fluids away from tissues that need them.

Post-event nutrition. This is a very important aspect to recovery that many kids overlook. The amount of energy spent needs to be replaced to allow the body to be ready for the next training session or exercise bout. Your child's muscles are like wide receivers just waiting to restore what they have used up. The ability to soak up muscle carbohydrate like a sponge is best during the first 30 to 60 minutes after exercise, and the process seems to work better with a little protein. This restoration process has important implications.

INSTANT REPLAY

A muscle's ability to soak up carbohydrates to replenish energy storage is best during the first 30 to 60 minutes after exercise.

If your child uses up more stored energy than she replaces, you can see that the storage unit will slowly get emptier over time. Inability to completely and properly replenish carbohydrate stores can lead to a progressive decline in performance, exercise staleness, overtraining, depression, and immune system malfunction. Nutritional sources are not only important for carbohydrate replacement, but also for antioxidants that are critical for providing the clearing machinery necessary to get rid of free radicals and other chemical by-products of exercise and keep the immune system and other cells healthy.

Rehydration must also occur to make up for sweat losses and heat exposure. Remember that having a poor thirst drive is a developmental problem with youngsters. They also base their intake on taste. These characteristics show the importance of having mandatory drink breaks and also determining the best way for your child to want to have adequate fluid intake. Water is usually great, but kids often will not like it because it has no taste. It will suffice for short events, but if there are longer situations, your child may need something different to keep her adequately hydrated. Some of the electrolyte sports drinks taste better to them, which helps them drink more, and those drinks also help keep the thirst drive stimulated because of the electrolyte effects.

The basic 4 components of performance are genetics, equipment, training and technique, and nutrition. Because genetics cannot be controlled and equipment can be equalized, it boils down to training and nutrition, which are intimately connected. Your youngster may train for hours, but without the right nutrition, training cannot be supported optimally. Kids have the added need to provide calories for both growth and exercise energy. Good nutrition is not limited by age and developmental boundaries, so proper nutritional practices can and should be started from birth.

INSTANT REPLAY

Kids have the added need to provide calories for both growth and exercise energy.

Every day I hear more about the worsening nutritional world that surrounds our youth, and every day I see, read, and hear more about the importance of fruits, vegetables, and grains for disease prevention and long-term health. So, Mom was always right. Back to the basics again. The government even thinks they are so important for disease prevention that it has raised the recommended daily servings and supports a new food pyramid. It's easy to recommend, but not always so easy to do. These basics apply to everyone. If youth are to grow and exercise properly, it's necessary for them to eat properly—but they don't. Kids and adults can be pretty picky and not only have trouble getting the daily recommended servings, but getting the variety they need to provide the most nutritionally intense value of food. If that is difficult, it's nice to know that there are helpful solutions to getting some of that valuable nutrition by using whole-food fruits and vegetables in capsules in addition to their daily food intake. Of the various encapsulated food products available, the one I happen to recommend to my patients and athletes is Juice Plus+ because of its extensive independent medical research. It is always most important to get the best nutrition from food first and foremost because it also provides calories for growth and sustaining exercise. I always encourage youngsters to eat more whole-food fruits, vegetables, grains, and healthy fats instead of sugary or trans fat snacks. The benefit is that many of those foods also serve as sources of good carbohydrates for exercise fuel, fighting the oxidative stress of exercise, and replenishing carbohydrate storage after exercise.

Application

When dealing with the pressures of training and competition, it is important to know there are many variables that affect performance, such as genetics, development, and emotional maturity. Yet nutrition is a major component that is too often overlooked for its benefits of providing energy and chemical protection for optimal performance. Sometimes it is easy to focus on the activity itself without realizing that proper food intake can also play a foundational role in how well that activity is carried out. Youngsters are developmentally unique in the way they handle thirst and the fact that their bodies require nutrition for growth and activity at the same time. It may be helpful for you to enlist the aid of a nutritionist to give you a better ballpark idea of the magnitude of calories your child will need. It will probably surprise you. Understanding the benefits of good nutrition and its importance for protecting the body from the chemicals produced from exercise stress and providing fuel for optimal participation and fuel replacement will be just one more way to maximize the sports and activity experience. Nutrition is fuel for your child. Fuel for your teenager. Fuel for champions at any level.

★ ★ ★ ★ ★ ★ ★ ★ ★ ★ ★ ★ ★ ★ ★ ★

SUCCESS RX

1. You should approach supplement use in your child with great hesitancy because potential or actual side effects are unknown for actively growing bodies and there is very little research to support the claims.

2. Fruits and vegetables contain vitamins in natural form that are combined with thousands of plant chemicals and enzymes, all of which work together to help the body effectively and efficiently use them.

3. Ways to reduce oxidative stress and free radical production from exercise include spreading out highly intense exercise, allowing sufficient recovery time and adequate rest, staying well hydrated, and having daily nutrition that is high in antioxidants.

4. The ability of a muscle to replace carbohydrate stores is best during the first 30 to 60 minutes after exercise.

5. In youth, tremendous calories are required to grow and build important body tissues as well as fuel exercise demands. Proper nutritional sources are not only important for carbohydrate replacement and energy supply, but also for antioxidants for clearing free radicals and other chemical by-products of exercise while keeping the immune system and other cells healthy.

6. Youngsters are developmentally unique in the way they handle thirst and the fact that their bodies require nutrition for growth and activity at the same time.

★ ★ ★ ★ ★ ★ ★ ★ ★ ★ ★ ★ ★ ★ ★ ★

Between You and Me

1. Your child may be bombarded with suggestions for the latest supplement fad. Be careful. It is difficult to think of any significant reason a growing child would need any type of performance-enhancing substance, especially when they are not scientifically researched for children, if at all. How can you redirect your youngster toward the benefits of good nutrition as another way to improve his or her activity?

2. Kids usually don't have a good thirst drive, so waiting to drink fluids once they are thirsty isn't going to be enough. How can you help ensure your youngster is staying adequately hydrated?

3. Proper nutrition is our main source of exercise fuel. It is also important to protect from the production of oxidative stress, provide for growth of healthy tissues, and aid in restoring and refueling energy storage. All are critical for optimal functioning. What are good food sources your child will eat to help with both aspects?

Pump Up the Volume

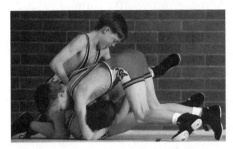

Ho hum. What to do? Guess I'll see what's on TV.

Click…no. No. Cartoons. More cartoons. MTV. Nope. Cooking channel. No way. Ah! ESPN. What's this? The Mr Teenage Bodybuilding contest. Gee! These kids are just a few years older than I am? Wow. They must have been lifting weights for a long time.

OK. Enough of that. Maybe I will just go outside and play with our dog.

Hey, the mail came! Junk mail, lots of bills for Mom and Dad, Sports Illustrated *for my brother, some fitness magazine for my sister, more bills, and more bills. Man, these people in these magazines must exercise all the time! I guess everybody looks this way. So how come I don't? Am I OK? Maybe in a few years….*

Mom! Glad you're back. It was boring around here. Hey, Mom, when can I start lifting weights?

Somehow, something got lost in translation when muscles changed from being used for gathering food to being a way of life and look. It is so standard to look a certain way that strength is not always an issue; simply how you appear seems most important. Young kids are exposed to the "beautiful people" so much that it is normal now for junior high and high school boys to pump weights and shave their body to get that magazine-model look. Until a decade ago, those rituals were reserved for those involved in bodybuilding and swimming (the price to pay for wearing a Speedo). But now, appearance is so paramount that kids want muscles—just because!

It is astonishing to know what is going on in our schools. The use of anabolic steroids is increasing to levels we don't even know among junior high and high school students. Some are athletes succumbing to the pressure of doing anything to win. Some are not athletes at all, but use such dangerous drugs just to look good. Go figure. Who could imagine that young teens addicted to steroids would become the cover article of *Newsweek?* This is a terrible situation that is growing out of hand. The news frequently shows prominent sports figures and teams getting in trouble with steroid scandals. Youngsters rarely know the side effects and as usual, even if they do, they think the bad things will never happen to them. Desiring muscles for more strength and power, athletic superiority, or even a ripped body is not necessarily abnormal. However, if the desired end result is one built from pressure to perform, a distortion of what a healthy body really is, or a disregard for personal safety, that is a problem. Some youth think muscles are the answer to everything, and they will go to dangerous lengths to develop them.

Other youth just see muscles all around them and think they should have them to avoid being different. Muscles are important, but they are not the end all and be all for participating in activities or sports. There is so much more that contributes to the complete package of improving sports skills and expertise. We have been discussing all of the different factors that develop over time to benefit ability. Strength is just one of them.

INSTANT REPLAY

There are so many things that develop over time to contribute to the complete package of improving sports skills and expertise—strength is just one of them.

Let's put the steroid craze and muscle mania aside and talk about strength training as it applies and contributes to your child's various sporting endeavors and how development plays a part. So what about lifting weights? It may be easy to think that the sooner your child starts lifting weights, the quicker he will be able to run faster, jump higher, and throw farther. Well, think again. Maybe that is why none of the infant stores carry any beginner baby weight sets in pink and blue. When considering the question of when Johnny can start lifting weights, there are several issues that must be addressed. Among the more important issues are

- Age
- Level of development
- Reason for interest

- Level of sports skill already achieved
- Risk of injury
- Availability of equipment and adequate supervision
- Reality of gaining strength (and size)
- How strength training works in a young body

Age and Level of Development

The importance of age would appear to even the most casual observer to be a no-brainer. Alas, you do not see some of the patients in my medical practice. You would be amazed how many parents are frothing at the mouth to have their kids lifting weights at very young ages or when they have just started a new sport. Whoa! Hang on a bit. To add a little reality to the scenario of prepubertal iron pumping, let's look at the reality of science and research. This isn't *Dumbbells for Dummies* here. I'm talking scientific research, and there has actually been a lot of scientific interest in this subject. Inquiring minds want to know if it's OK for young Johnny or Janie to be reaching for those weights.

Many years ago, people abandoned the notion of youth lifting weights altogether. The thought was that children were not able to get stronger or bigger because they did not have enough testosterone in their bodies until after puberty. We have learned a lot since then and now know that girls and boys can actually gain strength before they are even close to puberty. The real question is not how that happens, but is it necessary or even worth it? I will discuss with you how it happens and things to consider when deciding if it is necessary or appropriate.

Age is a big factor. To carry out strength training effectively, athletes must have correct form and be able to move the weight in a safe and efficient manner. We have seen in earlier chapters that balance control, posture, and coordination start to mature to adult levels by around 7 to 8 years of age. In the majority of cases, it would not be appropriate (or safe) to allow weight training before age 7. It still seems to be common sense that strength training even at that age is questionable for any long-term benefit. Other developmental factors play a role here, too. Milestones such as attention span, ability to stay focused, and maturity to accept and understand instruction all apply. If the child has not reached a level of development to satisfy those criteria, spend the time and energy doing something else and let him lift the garbage instead of weights.

INSTANT REPLAY

It is important for mature balance control to have developed prior to considering a strength training program.

Reason for Interest

When I am confronted with the question, "Can my child lift weights?" I often revert to my childhood and respond with a simple, "Why?" It is often quite apparent who is behind the reason for the interest. If the child has no interest or is not ready, the game is over. If it seems all the interest is from the parents or coaching staff, I must investigate why they think it is so important. Remember, kids want to have fun. If Johnny or Julie is not interested, forcing the issue rarely leads to a positive or successful activity experience.

On the other hand, if your youngster has a genuine desire and interest to proceed with a strength training program, the question should be taken seriously and the entire situation should be evaluated. This still does not mean it will be appropriate after all the factors have been investigated, but consideration is a good place to start. If the genuine reason is just to look good in surf shorts at 9 years of age, forget it. Hormones have to be there to allow the muscles to grow significantly. If the genuine reason is to accentuate strength for an activity or sport in which your child is involved, and he has reached some of the important developmental milestones necessary to carry out a strengthening program, it is legitimate to at least discuss it further.

Level of Sports Skill Already Achieved

Sometimes youth will hear that older athletes have improved or won an event because they started lifting weights. These youth rarely realize that the older athlete was also going through puberty and was getting stronger anyway. If athletes have the desire, motivation, and the appropriate developmental milestones and already achieved a certain level of skill in their sports activity, strength training may complement and enhance their participation. Remember, just being stronger at something does not necessarily make one better! Bigger, stronger muscles won't make your child a sensational hockey player if the skills to play hockey are not there in the first place. Strength is just one piece of the big performance puzzle. If the youngster is barely skilled in the sport, strength training is probably not appropriate.

Why get stronger at something you are not good at yet? It hardly makes sense.

INSTANT REPLAY

If a youngster is barely skilled in a sport or activity, strength training is probably not appropriate until it can be applied to more improved skill development.

On the flip side, it may be appropriate when the child has already mastered many of the basic and transitional skills of the sport, has already achieved some noticeable accomplishment and improvement, wants to supplement overall training with some sports-specific strength training, and is not being pressured to be involved with weights.

Risk of Injury

Strength training must be approached with caution and respect. Weights cannot be taken lightly (no pun intended). Old wives' tales used to suggest that strength training would "stunt your growth." This could easily happen if there is a major accident that injures the growth plate because it is the weakest area of the bone. Beyond speculation, though, there have been sufficient reports of major injuries to withhold kids from training with weights. Unfortunately, some of those injuries have been deaths. Most of the serious injuries have come from situations with home gym equipment when there was no supervision and the kids were playing around or challenging one another. This problem may not apply to youth teams, but even so, this type of dangerous situation simply must not happen. Youngsters should be taught from the beginning that playing with such equipment is a big no-no, like playing with sharp knives or guns. Not only can they put an eye out, but someone can get seriously hurt. Most of the reported injuries involve unsupervised situations or youth attempting to do a max lift before they are physically developed or have the right instruction.

INSTANT REPLAY

Strength training must be approached with caution and respect.

Most reported serious injuries involve unsupervised situations or youth attempting a max lift before they are physically developed or have the right instruction.

Injuries have included herniated disks in the back, muscle strains and tears, bone fractures, growth plate injuries, and cartilage damage. If lifting weights is going to be pursued seriously, that type of training should be pursued in the right way and correctly along the developmental pathway. The American Academy of Pediatrics recommends that explosive types of lifts or heavy Olympic-style lifting should be delayed until the skeleton matures after the growth spurt.

In general, training with weights has been found to help increase strength in children without negative effects on things such as bone growth or blood pressure. Outside the realm of unsupervised home gym equipment, proper strength training has been shown to allow an increase in strength with fewer injuries than occur during recess at school. This does not mean that there is no risk. Risk is always present and potentially high, but risk can be reduced significantly if strength training is done appropriately. For young age groups before puberty, this means doing light weights with more repetitions. It also means strengthening sports-specific moves and actions to better equip the child in those positions. Overall flexibility should be emphasized as well because a little momentum for maintaining flexibility is needed before youngsters start to tighten up with the rapid growth of puberty.

Availability of Equipment and Adequate Supervision

These 2 external factors play a significant role in the safety of strength training for kids. If the equipment is not readily available, is not the right kind of equipment, or is in an unsupervised setting, participation in that location should be reconsidered. Most gym equipment is made for adult-sized bodies, so it is too big for kids; the arm and leg lengths are too long, and the weight plates increase a large amount at a time. Fortunately, machines that are built in sizes for children do exist in some places, but are certainly not widespread. In that case, free weights can often be used more safely and effectively because they are readily available and portable, can replicate many different sports-specific moves and positions, and can start out very small and only increase by a small amount of weight at a time. Of course, good, mature posture and balance control are absolutely necessary before starting to use free weights.

In addition, low-weight, higher-repetition exercises need to be done correctly. Proper form and technique must be strictly guided and supervised by a trained certified professional or coach who has knowledge about strength training for children. This is of enormous importance. Supervision is not an older high school student who just passes through the gym every now and then during his free period. Supervision means a knowledgeable adult who has devoted time to help teach proper form and observe the child to prevent injury. Because of the high risk of dangerous injury, lifting heavy weights with bad technique and bad supervision is only asking for disaster. Even when done properly with appropriate supervision, an injury can happen, but the many scientific studies investigating strength training in 8- to 11-year-olds show that injury rates have been virtually nonexistent when training is done correctly with strict supervision. Are you getting the picture here? The word *supervision* was used 5 times in just 1 paragraph. It must be important. Let me say it again. Regardless of development or sports expertise, strength training for young people must be carried out with correct technique and strict supervision. One word, 4 syllables—sounds like *supervision.*

INSTANT REPLAY

Regardless of development or sports expertise, strength training for young people must be carried out with correct technique and strict supervision.

Reality of Gaining Strength (and Size) and How Strength Training Works in a Young Body

So after all this hoopla, what is the chance that a 9-year-old can actually get stronger by training with weights? When looking at the results of more than 30 well-done scientific studies on the subject, the evidence is there. Before puberty, kids can gain significant strength without stunting their growth or even getting big muscles. Different types of scans have revealed no significant change in muscle size in children who have not yet reached puberty, but strength is increased. How is that possible? The body is an amazing machine, as we are all finding out. When these young muscles are challenged, impulses from nerves recruit more muscle fibers into action. This increased muscle fiber activation allows children to increase strength over a period of training that usually needs to be at least 8 weeks long. Most of this research has been performed using youth who are not on sports teams, so the increased recruitment of muscle fibers may be different for a youngster who is at a higher level of training and using more muscle fibers already.

INSTANT REPLAY

Before puberty, girls and boys can gain significant strength without stunting growth or getting big muscles.

Strength is gained by increased nerve recruitment of muscle fibers.

So you just asked if your child can lift weights. This has been a long answer to a short question. Now you know why. Shouldn't it be a straight yes or no answer? Obviously not. Is it *possible* to lift weights? Sure. Is it really *appropriate?* Maybe. Is it actually *necessary?* Let's look at the whole scenario before deciding if the light is green to go ahead with a strength training program. It's like looking both ways before crossing a really busy street. There are so many factors that play a role in determining whether strength training is safe, appropriate, and purposeful for your child. My goal in this chapter was to explain those factors so you can have more knowledge for better decisions. Better decisions for positive experiences. Positive experiences for reality sports success.

★ ★ ★ ★ ★ ★ ★ ★ ★ ★ ★ ★ ★ ★ ★ ★

SUCCESS RX

1. Girls and boys can gain strength well before puberty, but developmental considerations must be taken into account prior to engaging in a strengthening program. There are many factors that play a role in determining whether strength training is safe, appropriate, and purposeful for your child.

2. It may be appropriate to begin a strengthening program when the child has already mastered many of the basic and transitional skills of the sport, has already achieved some noticeable accomplishment and improvement, wants to supplement overall training with some sports-specific strength training, and is not being pressured to be involved with weights.

3. The risk for injury is potentially high, but can be reduced significantly if training is done with correct technique and strict supervision.

★ ★ ★ ★ ★ ★ ★ ★ ★ ★ ★ ★ ★ ★ ★ ★

Between You and Me

1. Maybe you have discussed strength training with your child, or someone else has brought it up. Maybe your child has mentioned it out of the blue at the dinner table. In either case, what is the real reason your child wants to lift weights?

2. Your child is engaged in recreational activities, but seems insistent about going to a gym and has a new interest in getting bigger and stronger. This may be normal for the age and activity level of the child, but it may also be very out of character. Is he being pushed from other sources?

3. If all the cards are in the deck, development has progressed, skills have been accomplished, and self-improvement has been substantial, then strength training may be appropriate for your child, depending on the desire that is present. What is a fun way to mix in a little strength training as part of your child's overall exercise program and not make it the central focus?

Prescription for Success

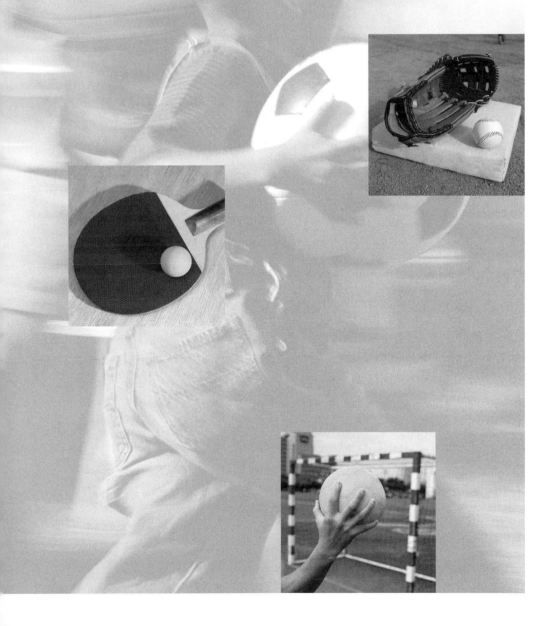

Coaches Huddle

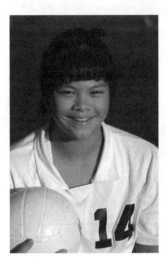

That was a good race. I didn't win, but I feel good about what I did. I corrected some mistakes from last time and gave it all I could! Last time, I was really bummed, but this time, I am happy with my performance. A lot of it comes from my coach making me realize that winning is way more than coming in first. If I give my best effort on that day, focus on using my best technique, don't give up, and congratulate my opponent, I have been a winner that time. Sounds a lot more fun to me! I like that because I can be a winner a lot more often than if I just get first place every now and then.

Gimme a W! Gimme an I! You know the rest of the drill. What's it spell? Well, let's talk about redefining that big little word *win*. Redefining takes a huge effort and is a drastic change from what society thinks—and more importantly, a drastic change from what we think! Patterns and thought processes are hard to redirect after they have been established for years. Webster's may have only a few definitions of the word, but life defines winning in many ways. Redefining winning automatically redefines success.

Every adult, sibling, and peer has the chance to instill a healthy definition of reality success into active youth. Probably many of you with past experience as an athlete can acknowledge that one of the most influential figures shaping the young athletic mind is—the envelope please—the coach. Coaches usually take the Oscar with the parents securing Best Supporting Actor. Most coaches are incredibly deserving of this honor (although some win for playing the role of the evil villain). Good coaches need to be applauded. They not only have a major duty of teaching, instructing, and coaching kids day in and day out, but also spend an amazing amount of time traveling to competitions and living much of their lives poolside, on the field, at the track, by the court, or on the mat. Many children and adolescents spend more time with coaches than family, so coaches often fulfill a parental role as well and can become substantial role models. Nothing makes a person gain more respect for the coaching or parenting profession than when you are placed in that situation. I was a coach of sorts at many sports camps and realized I loved being coached more than being one. There are a lot of serious responsibilities wrapped up in the role of coach. So when you find a great one, show that coach your respect. The coach is worth it.

Alas, I digress. I will never forget trying many different sports as a child and being downright poor at most of them, and I will remember my literal first plunge into the pool of sports being anything but

glamorous. When I broke my elbow and was instructed to swim
as therapy, my mom found the new swim coach in the community.
I trotted right out on the pool deck thinking it would be no sweat.
I mean, come on, I had spent many days playing around in the local
community pool. Well, I had to think again. I dove in to swim one
length of the pool, got halfway, thought I was going to drown, and
stopped. Choking, gasping, spitting water everywhere—great, another
failed attempt, I thought. The coach stood there nodding and said,
"Yep. Look's like we've got a long way to go. [*Very long silence.*] Better
get started tomorrow." My heart jumped! He thinks I can do this! I will
never know if I was truly genetically suited for swimming, but knowing my coach and parents believed in me made all the difference in
the world and took me from an early failure to a college All-American
to a nationally ranked masters swimmer. Bravo, Coach. Bravo, Mom
and Dad. You may not have done the swimming for me, but you
sure made it easier and more desirable for me to put in the effort.

Unfortunately, many of my fellow swimmers on other teams
didn't fare so well and quit forever after being pushed to physical and
emotional burnout over the years. Sadly, this scenario is happening in
many sports activities to our participating kids and teens more often
than it should—which is *never*. Coaches and parents may not realize
the tremendous impact they have, but face it—they do. You may
already be a coach who makes exercise, sports, and activities enjoyable experiences. You may be eager to be one. Hopefully you care,
because *your* child is being coached by someone.

So what can a coach do to provide a positive experience? Coaches
are knowledgeable about activities and sports, but must continue

to be knowledgeable about the kids they are coaching. Learning about the unique differences in children and teenagers and the enormous variability among them can make a huge difference in coaching college softball versus coaching softball for 9-year-olds. Remember the many developmental, chemical, and mental aspects of kids and how these aspects affect their ability to learn and play recreational activities and sports of any level. Lack of this knowledge, not understanding that knowledge, or failing to use that understanding can lead to an unsuccessful and stressful experience.

INSTANT REPLAY

Coaches are knowledgeable about activities and sports, but must continue to be knowledgeable about the kids they are coaching.

Take the developmental aspects, for instance. Knowing *why* a 5- or 6-year-old needs to hit a stationary ball is valuable to reduce outside pressure on the child while allowing the child to have a positive experience and sense of accomplishment. Having a good handle on the developmental milestones and their sequence of maturation will enable a coach to provide for more achievements by making appropriate adjustments in playing time, equipment, instruction style, and approach to certain skills. Help guarantee the chances for reality sports success by giving kids smaller tasks to learn and accomplish. Show enthusiasm! Kids are sometimes like pets—they can detect genuineness and good character. So make the experience one in which the kids feel comfortable and unafraid to try new skills.

INSTANT REPLAY

Having a good handle on the developmental milestones and their sequence of maturation will enable a coach to provide for more achievements.

Understanding the chemical differences in youth can allow focus on skill development without the unnecessary addition of training time that may just lead to injury. Use caution in warmer environments and make them take breaks to drink fluids. Guide them in proper nutrition. Realize that kids are not small adults and that training youngsters with intense adult training programs is not only inappropriate, but also potentially unsafe. Increased overuse injuries can decrease training time or even end a promising career. If your goal is to have optimal time to train and teach youth, give them the chance to respond 100% effectively rather than only 60% because of an injury; that does not help you, the coach, or the child participant to maximize potential. Supervise all weight training efforts and only recommend such training if the athlete has reached an appropriate level of skill achievement and discipline.

Seeing how to approach a youngster from a psychological standpoint not only enables the child to gain self-confidence and self-esteem, but also can provide the bonus of coaching a youngster to success in many ways. Make statements that are rewarding, yet sincere. Find more things to compliment than condemn, and especially give attention and reward to the child's effort. Then constructive *correction* (notice I did not say criticism) is more apt to be received with a genuine desire to do better. It is critical to have realistic expectations and communicate with the child. Keeping athletes based in reality along their progression can help protect them from the stresses of unrealistic expectations thrown at them from the rest of the world.

Be alert to the causes of burnout and strive to keep the athlete motivated and interested with positive feedback. Excessive demands physically and emotionally and on time management can overload the youngster. As athletes progress to higher levels of training and competition, they need to have foundational input on what it means to win or lose. Winning should not be overemphasized, and losing should be seen as opportunity to improve. Disappointment is normal, but feeling fear caused by failure can jeopardize a young athlete's ability to maximize potential.

INSTANT REPLAY

Winning should not be overemphasized, and losing should be seen as an opportunity to improve.

Desired characteristics of youth coaches include helping kids have fun, focusing on teaching skills, emphasizing good sportsmanship, placing attention on achievement rather than winning, verbally supporting accomplishments, and developing a concept of true reality success that goes way beyond crossing the finish line first. Poor coaching uses negative feedback, intimidation, criticism, or demeaning discipline.

INSTANT REPLAY

Desired characteristics of youth coaches include helping kids have fun, focusing on teaching skills, emphasizing good sportsmanship, placing attention on achievement rather than winning, verbally supporting accomplishments, and developing a concept of true reality success that goes way beyond crossing the finish line first.

Remember what surveys show—kids want to have fun and play more, no matter if they win or lose. So make sure the activity is geared toward having fun. When working with young children, let every child participate as equally as possible, no matter the level of talent on the rest of the team. Sometimes that takes a dose of difficult pride-swallowing, like the circus guy who somehow gets a flaming sword down his throat. There are also times when a coach does everything right, treats every youngster equally and fairly, and yet still has to dodge verbal bullets from parents like a charging bull— olé! Keeping calm and sticking to the plan is commendable—many pats on the back for that. Coaching involves acts of unselfishness and placing as a top priority the goal of helping kids develop a healthy view of exercise and activities. You have the chance to positively affect their future participation for life. I can personally vouch for that. Believe me, the satisfaction and recognition a coach can get from such acts may be as meaningful as a league championship.

One of the many benefits to come from exercise activity besides general health is the formation of a healthy self-esteem and sense of self-accomplishment. Anything you can do as a coach to foster that process will be worth its weight in gold. Kids tend to model adults they respect, so passing on a positive approach is a truly valuable inheritance. If you're a coach who is in it for the glory and fame, stick with adult athletics. If it matters to leave a legacy and help a youngster learn skills that affect her outlook on exercise and life, come on in, the water's fine. The world of youth sports awaits.

★ ★ ★ ★ ★ ★ ★ ★ ★ ★ ★ ★ ★ ★ ★ ★ ★

SUCCESS RX

What Coaches Can Do to Create a Positive Youth Sports Experience

- Redefine success.

- Be knowledgeable about the sport you are coaching.

- Be knowledgeable about the age group you are coaching.

- Understand the unique developmental skill patterns of that age group and make adjustments for that skill level.

- Remember that the inability to perform a certain skill may just be a lack of developmental timing, rather than a true lack of ability.

- Reinforce and refine the skills that are achieved without pushing too quickly for other skills.

- Give kids small tasks to learn to increase chances for accomplishment.

- Be enthusiastic and genuine.

- Make kids feel comfortable so they are not afraid to try new skills.

- Let everyone play and substitute players frequently.

- Focus your verbal support on what skills they do right. Then your coaching support can more easily be directed at making constructive corrections in other skills.

- Understand chemical development so you do not train a child like an adult, risking overtraining and injury.

- Know the limitations of aerobic development so you can maintain a solid aerobic base without overtraining, and concentrate on technique.

- Use caution in warmer conditions and hot environments and take frequent water breaks.

- Know when the circumstances are appropriate for weight training.

- Make your rewarding statements sincere.

- Have realistic expectations and communicate them so the active youngster can see improvement and acknowledge accomplishment more frequently and be more protected from societal pressure to perform for an ultimate prize.

- Be alert for signs of overtraining and burnout.

- Keep kids motivated with positive feedback.

- Remember the importance of positive effects on early psychological development.

- As kids progress, give meaningful input on winning and losing and emphasize that every practice and competition is an opportunity to learn and improve.

- Teach how to learn from successes, disappointments, and everything in between.

- Do not coach by intimidation.

- Be a good role model.

- Instill good sportsmanship (they are watching your example).

- Teach good fundamental skills that the child can use to build on with the next coach or activity.

- Foster a sense of self-worth and confidence in the child or teen.

- Emphasize effort and accomplishment more than winning.

- Gear the activity toward fun and a positive experience. You may be the very coach that helps inspire a child to stay involved in a sport and truly maximize his or her potential for reality success.

★ ★ ★ ★ ★ ★ ★ ★ ★ ★ ★ ★ ★ ★ ★

Between You and Me

1. Sometimes it is difficult for a parent or child to have any choice when it comes to coaches. If you can be selective, have you thought about what characteristics you should look for in a coach?

2. It can be easy to have an approach to coaching that is your particular style. Sometimes, that style may not be "one style fits all." If you are a coach, how can you build on your coaching style and occasionally individualize it with kids to make the experience a pleasant and unforgettable one?

3. Now you are more informed about the effect of development on skills for sports and exercise activities. What new things can you say and do, based on the different levels of development, that will make the activity fun, give the kids a sense of accomplishment, and boost self-esteem?

Your Child Is Not You

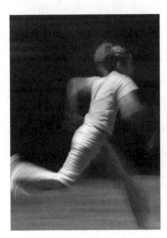

Some of my friends are so fun to play sports with, and others are so not cool. We just look at things differently. Sometimes I just don't get it. I thought everybody had a family like mine.

I love it when I am so thrilled after a practice or event and my parents say, "We are so proud of you for doing your best." It's great, too, when I am bummed and upset and my parents say, "We are so proud of you for doing your best." And they are not just repeating themselves—they really mean it each time in different ways! It just makes me try as hard as I can, knowing they won't think different of me if I win or lose.

The only thing I don't love is that when I do win, I still have to help with the dishes!

Parenting. Wow. Isn't it amazing how much is crammed into those 9 little letters? Family responsibilities. Schools. Parent-teacher meetings. Homework. Music lessons. Band concerts. Choir. School clubs. Sports games. Weekend games. Practices. Chauffeur. Chef. Clothes shopping. Grocery shopping. Breakfast. Lunch. Dinner. Snacks. Laundry. More snacks. Financial support. Future college education. Mentoring. Modeling. Listening. Discipline. Encouragement. Caring. Support. Love. And the list goes on and on and on. And if everyday responsibilities aren't enough, we have easily become a society of overcommitment. Sometimes families become so activity oriented that they have less valuable time for the responsibilities of raising their children to be caring, kind, independent, responsible, and contributing adults. Life simply becomes the next carpool to the next sports activity. Parents who juggle commitments with responsibilities like they're in Cirque de Soleil get major kudos. They seem to be able to maintain a balance between importance for the moment versus importance for the long haul.

Often adults learn little about being a parent until they become one. Nothing like being thrown into the fire! There is not always a lot of help except doing what your parents did, talking to your parents to see how you acted, or talking to your friends who have already swung their machete through the parenting jungle. Everyone is looking for *the* instruction manual, *the* parts list, *the* rule book. Sometimes that is the beauty of life; some of the rules are made up as we go along. But along that path it is helpful to have some general direction and guidance. I hope to add some of that direction to help you and your child approach sports and activities with more understanding and confidence. You may want your child just to be active. You may want to your kid to be a standout. You may want your teen to be a college star.

You may want your youngster to go pro. You may want all of that— and want it *now.*

Have patience. Any good refining process takes time. If too many steps in the process are skipped, the end result will be lacking. Does this, by chance, bring back any humorous memories of the frantic nighttime holiday assembly of Johnny's or Julie's coveted gift that happened to have 347 pieces and a 24-page instruction booklet? In a very simple way, think of your wonderful living gift as one of those long-term projects under construction. Assembly is required; batteries are included. Each year more nuts and bolts of skills get added to the beginning genetic foundation. You may get to tighten some of the screws yourself. Other parts are more fixed or cannot be tightened until other parts have already been assembled. Knowing about the process can help the final construction be as sturdy as possible without as much risk of someone bulldozing the house down.

You want your kid to have an advantage over the other kids? Learn about the decathlon of development and think of ways to support the process of skill acquisition without excessive pressure or unrealistic expectations. That may be just the opposite of what you may think, but pushing too hard may delay some of the natural acquisition of skills and maturation of self-confidence and thus defeat your goal of having an advantage. There are definitely kids who have a ton of talent, but cannot produce because they lack the self-confidence to succeed. They have too much pressure from their parents or are coached with intimidation, so they choose the path of least resistance to avoid conflict, perform just enough without risking failure, and never reach their full potential. Remember, your child is uniquely different than you, so living vicariously through your active child to satisfy your needs can be extremely dangerous. In addition, there are definitely kids who are not as talented, but are totally accomplished because their parents and coaches give them a support structure that allows them to try, fail, learn, grow, try again, accomplish, and succeed. There it is again—reality success.

So what can a parent do to replace the word *pressure* with the word *positive* or the word *stress* with the word *success?* No one can guarantee an Olympic medal for that youngster of yours, but parents can help increase maximum potential by following a few simple suggestions. Most importantly, support for your child must be unconditional. Children must know that their worth and value is unrelated to winning or their performance. They should be praised for learning a new skill, mastering a certain technique, giving a great effort, and of course, winning if they work hard and earn first place. Credit given for credit due. If he improves in high school basketball, hallelujah. If she gets Olympic skiing gold, fantastic. They both deserve their own success that is their personal reality. Find things to praise even if there are few, and remember that disappointments should never be equated with failure. Start a new vocabulary that redefines success and includes reality success. Teach your child that winning includes many things besides a blue ribbon.

INSTANT REPLAY

Support for your child or teen must be unconditional and unrelated to his or her performance.

Start a new vocabulary that redefines success and includes reality success.

Know the developmental process and be patient to see the prize of new skills achieved. Understand what your youngster can do, when it can be done, and why you can't always do much to make it happen more quickly. Realize what skill level your child has reached and focus more on helping improve that skill than looking prematurely to the next skill that is not yet ready. Let me put it into perspective— that would be like opening a rosebud before it's ready…not a pretty sight. Crinkly petals. Muted color. Lack of fragrance. A flower is most beautiful when it opens at the right time in its developmental sequence. Is it really worth it to force the bud open too quickly? And what about picking a piece of fruit too early? Hard, dry, and poor taste. Ripening on the vine and picking it on time yields the most delicious result. Understanding the process will save you from a lot of unnecessary frustration and your child or teen from a lot of unnecessary performance anxiety. At the same time, it will enable both of you to enjoy the most positive experience possible.

INSTANT REPLAY

Realize what skill level your child has reached and focus more on helping improve that skill than looking prematurely to the next skill that is not yet ready.

Encourage your youngster any way you can. Build him up whether it is schoolwork, house chores, art projects, music performances, exercise, or sports. Kids need to hear and see you. It is important they hear your encouragement along with seeing you at the event for which they have worked hard to participate. This requires unselfishness with your time, but it will mean the world to your kid—and to his kids, someday. Keep your comments constructive. Comments should be encouraging and helpful without a lot of addenda and contingencies. Remember that positive statements eventually get lost if you get in the habit of always following a positive statement with, "Good job, *but...*"

Give your youngster a chance to take some responsibility for her sport, such as maintaining equipment, setting the alarm to get up for morning workouts (and you be the second wake-up call if the snooze alarm fails), or setting goals. At the same time, do not push her too much, or she will dread participating. Helping your child or teen set realistic, stepwise goals may also help your own personal expectations become more realistic. Goals that are too lofty without smaller interim goals along the way often increase the risk of burnout caused by lack of accomplishment and a feeling of incompetence. That happens if the only view of success is that final, ultimate, dream-come-true goal without any room for the many reality successes necessary to get there. Kids should never feel pressure to perform for parents apart from the normal stresses of competition. If more realistic goals are set, everyone can be happy when they are met. This achievement makes setting the next goals more exciting and meaningful.

Allow sports changes, if necessary. If the child has given a reasonable effort and attempt and wants to move on to something else, help him pursue something of his interest. Changing a sport is not a crime and often can be pivotal in allowing a child to blossom in a new activity. Help your child build a sense of identity and polish the many different facets that make him the diamond he is. Point out character qualities that make you proud. Help him realize he is a valuable human being first. Then, if Johnny becomes a world champion, it is important that he can say, "Wrestling is what I do, not who I am."

★ ★ ★ ★ ★ ★ ★ ★ ★ ★ ★ ★ ★ ★ ★ ★

SUCCESS RX
What Parents Can Do to Create a Positive Youth Sports Experience

- Support for your child must be unconditional.

- Be patient for the process, and enjoy it.

- Understand how the developmental progression works for sports skills.

- Be knowledgeable that many of the developmental milestones for sports skills cannot be accelerated beyond their natural limit.

- Realize that physical, chemical, and mental development all affect ability and all progress along different timetables.

- Support achievements as they occur. This will reduce pressure to achieve skills that are not quite ready.

- Remember, your child has his or her own likes and dislikes and should be able to participate without pressure to choose a certain activity.

- Remember that there are developmental patterns for chemical changes that allow your child to be able to progress in training intensity when it is time.

- Understand the extra changes that occur in the puberty transition from child to teenager.

- Don't overreact to normal developmental processes and changes that occur during puberty and may temporarily affect ability.

- Understand the profound developmental effect of a firm positive foundation of self-esteem on future performance and ability to handle competitive pressure.

- Redefine success and make sure performance disappointments are not seen as failures that the child might take personally.

- Teach your child that winning means a lot more than a gold medal (you first have to believe that yourself).

- Encourage your child any way you can.

- Find more things your child is doing right than things to criticize.

- Support by being visible at their events.

- Keep your comments positive without a lot of addenda or stipulations.

- Help your children take some responsibilities for their sport without making them feel overwhelmed with duties.

- Watch for warning signs of burnout or avoidance.

- Remember your child is a child, not a child-sized adult.

- Help your child set realistic goals (not your goals).

- Allow changes in sports, and encourage exposure to different sports.

- Instill a sense of value in exercise and fitness regardless of structured competition.

- Communicate sincerely and often with your child about his or her desires.

- Help your child build a strong sense of self-worth and identity that is not dependent on the sport itself or level of achievement.

- Provide positive momentum by celebrating reality successes as often as possible.

★ ★ ★ ★ ★ ★ ★ ★ ★ ★ ★ ★ ★ ★ ★

Between You and Me

1. Look beyond your child not picking up dirty clothes and picking his or her nose for a moment. What things can you identify that your child does right?

2. Knowing more about the bumpy course of skill development gives you better ability to watch skills unfold and support accomplishment. How can you best encourage your child or teen along the road of development?

3. Examine your heart and mind. What expectations do you have that might be unreasonable, and what expectations can you have that *are* reasonable?

4. Use the tools you now have for awareness of how children grow and become able to perform certain skills. How can you support without pushing too hard?

5. Think about the way you handle successes and disappointments. How can you reaffirm your love, support, and commitment no matter the final score of the game?

Cooldown—How Do You Spell Success?

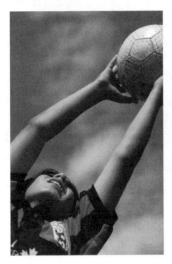

Congratulations! You did it. You have now officially been there, done that. You have finished what could potentially help your child travel on a road to maximum potential with fewer bumps along the way. Hopefully it is more comfortable to see how you can be there along the way to teach, guide, listen, support, protect, and encourage him or her to many episodes of reality sports success throughout life.

It is easy to dream big dreams for your kid, but keep those dreams in perspective. You may want Johnny or Julie to be a star, but pushing too much can injure a lot more than just an ankle. Coaches and parents have an awesome gift and responsibility to have youngsters under their care and guidance. Please make sure that guidance gives them a real sense of accomplishment and self-improvement, maximally develops their skills at an appropriate time and rate, and redefines the concepts of winning and success. That should help them self-achieve more than they ever could if under a lot of pressure.

INSTANT REPLAY

Please make sure that guidance gives your child a real sense of accomplishment and self-achievement, maximally develops his or her skills at an appropriate time and rate, and redefines the concepts of winning and success.

Let's rewind and recap for a moment. How in the world can parents have a million responsibilities and still be able to have a crystal ball telling them how their children develop into more active children and athletes of all different levels? They can't. That is why I spent 13 more years in school after high school. That is why I became a pediatrician. That is why I became a sports medicine specialist for children and teenagers.

Parents cannot possibly get all of this information from ESPN or *Ladies' Home Journal.* Concepts of sports development go way beyond the baby book basics. Does it really matter how sports skills develop after learning how to take those first few steps? You bet it does! There is so much importance in knowing when a child can balance well, hit a moving object, or run after a fly ball. Otherwise, coaches, parents, and young athletes alike can all become disillusioned and disappointed. This does not need to happen. Does understanding how aerobic fitness develops in your youngster matter? Of course it does! Refining technique and developing a good foundational aerobic base protects the child from overuse injuries and excessive miles of training before the body is ready. Is it a big deal to separate identity and self-worth from the sport or activity? Absolutely! The child has to be certain that her or his value as a human being comes from being loved unconditionally by you rather than from winning the race or game.

Youngsters are not small adults and have very specific and unique differences. With time and tons of education, our youth can take part in positive sports experiences with outcomes that are successful in many ways. It is obvious that only a small percentage of all athletes make it to the top of the medal stand, the best university, or the pros, so doesn't it make sense to help *all* children enjoy being active, see their skill improvements, maximize their potential, and enjoy small or large successes? If adults and children understand development and apply that understanding, they can enjoy their sports activities (no matter how high they rise), be more apt to continue to participate in some sort of exercise activity throughout their lives, maintain a positive health benefit, and be an example to their own children in the future. Put genetics aside for a minute. If you come from a phenomenal gene pool, you are fortunate. But those genetics do not guarantee success. Multiple factors from the outside play a significant role in how those genetics shine through from the inside. You should know how your child can accurately catch a crosscourt basketball as much as you know how many free throws he or she has made.

INSTANT REPLAY

If adults and children understand development and apply that understanding, they can enjoy their sports activites (no matter how high they rise), be more apt to continue being active throughout their lives, maintain health benefits, and be an example to their future children.

So congratulations to you. You have hopefully learned some new ideas and reinforced some old ones. I wish you new satisfaction in your outlook on youth activities and youth sports participation, like being handed the plate with the last chocolate chip cookie you baked. You get to enjoy the result of your creation and the fruits of your labor. Knowing a lot more about the intricacies of your child's development for activity participation is worth a lot. Knowing and understanding development to help you understand your child a lot better is priceless.

I wish you excitement as you finish this book and see how best to enable your young one to have a fantastic exposure to different activities and experience the success of achievement free of unnecessary pressure or injury. Pass the excitement on. Avoid being too competitive and share these pages with a neighbor. No, I am not suggesting everyone in the neighborhood gather around your kitchen table, hold hands, and sing Kumbayah. Think about the effects of multiplication—the potential for a better outcome for all involved is great if everyone has more knowledge and a healthier approach to exercise and youth sports. Having a better grip on all of this information allows you the confidence to watch your child or teen progress without being impatient or overreacting, which can reduce stress significantly.

Participation. All kids need to exercise their brains and bodies. Health problems, overweight, and health issues are problems in our society, and exercise needs to be encouraged for general overall health.

Practicality. Not all kids can win the gold or go pro, but all kids can have reality sports success at some level if we understand how to support them along their developmental road.

Protection. Kids need time to develop their skills, chemical balance, and psychological stamina. Overuse injuries are increasing because kids are pushing or being pushed too hard, too soon, too much, too quick.

Performance. Training and competition can be enjoyable and healthy activities for kids, parents, and coaches if approached with awareness, knowledge, patience, and unconditional support.

Respect the contributions from development and your contributions while it's happening.

Enjoy every achievement, large or small.

Accept differences in the abilities of youth.

Love your child no matter what athletic level is achieved.

Involve yourself, but allow space for your child to breathe.

Try many activities to see which ones click.

Yield your dreams and help your child form his or her own.

See the things your child does right.

Undo unrealistic expectations.

Communicate and learn your child's desires.

Conquer any desire to apply pressure.

Embrace your new knowledge of physical, chemical, and mental developmental skills.

Show that you care when your child triumphs and fails.

Support a new definition of success.

Many adults pressure youngsters or have unrealistic expectations because they don't possess helpful knowledge or information to make the correct approach or come up with reasonable expectations. But now you do. Apply it correctly and you may just see your child surpass what you thought would be his or her best potential. Priorities should be to provide your child with positive sports and activity experiences with as few pressures as possible and new definitions of success no matter the level. This attitude will affect future life achievements of your child as well as his or her lifelong approach to exercise and sports. I have enjoyed this; I hope you have, too. This is the kind of prescription I like writing—and do you know the best thing about this prescription? Unlimited refills. Come back as often as you like.

Development understood.
Improvement appreciated.
Skills not rushed.
Accomplishments made.
Progress rewarded.
Reality successes like these can occur daily for your child.

Maximize potential.
Minimize pressure.
Sports success R_x.
Your child's prescription for the best experience!

GO TEAM!

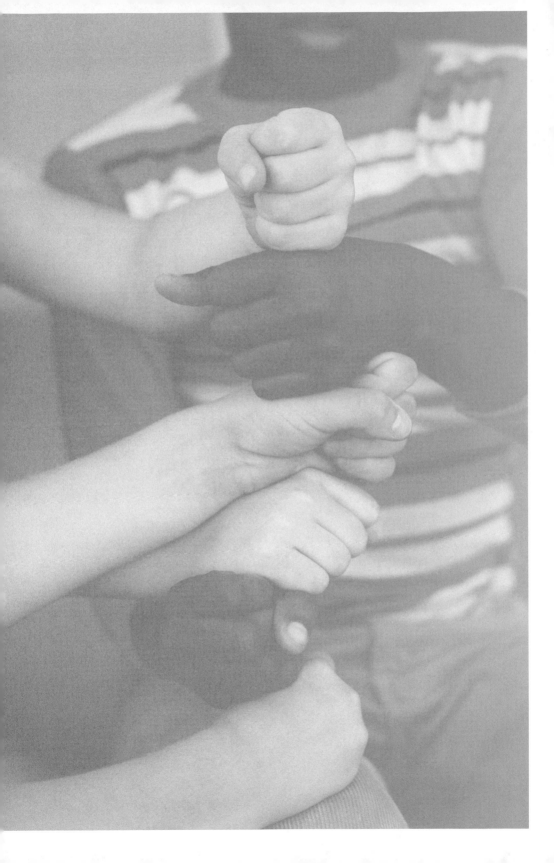

Index